THE TRUTH ABOUT
FAMILY LIFE

THE TRUTH ABOUT FAMILY LIFE

SECOND EDITION

Robert N. Golden, M.D.
University of Wisconsin-Madison
General Editor

Fred L. Peterson, Ph.D.
University of Texas-Austin
General Editor

Mark J. Kittleson, Ph.D., William Kane, Ph.D.,
and Richelle Rennegarbe, Ph.D.
Advisers to the First Edition

Amber Barnes, M.P.H., and Julia A. Watkins, Ph.D., M.P.H.
Principal Authors

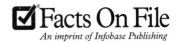
Facts On File
An imprint of Infobase Publishing

The Truth About Family Life, Second Edition

Facts On File, Inc.
An imprint of Infobase Publishing
132 West 31st Street
New York NY 10001

Library of Congress Cataloging-in-Publication Data

Barnes, Amber.
  The truth about family life / Amber Barnes and Julia Watkins, principal authors ; Robert N. Golden, general editor, Fred L. Peterson, general editor ; Mark J. Kittleson, William Kane and Richelle Rennegarbe, advisers to the first edition. − 2nd ed.
      p. cm.
  Originally entered under author: Renée Despres.
  Includes bibliographical references and index.
  ISBN-13: 978-0-8160-7641-3 (hardcover : alk. paper)
  ISBN-10: 0-8160-7641-3 (hardcover : alk. paper) 1. Families−United States. 2. Teenagers−Family relationships−United States. I. Watkins, Julia. II. Golden, Robert N. III. Peterson, Fred L. IV. Despres, Renée. Truth about family life. V. Title.
  HQ536.D43 2011
  306.85'0973'03−dc22
                                    2010049240

Facts On File books are available at special discounts when purchased in bulk quantities for businesses, associations, institutions, or sales promotions. Please call our Special Sales Department in New York at (212) 967-8800 or (800) 322-8755.

You can find Facts On File on the World Wide Web at http://www.factsonfile.com

Excerpts included herewith have been reprinted by permission of the copyright holders; the author has made every effort to contact copyright holders. The publishers will be glad to rectify, in future editions, any errors or omissions brought to their notice.

Text design by David Strelecky
Composition by Kerry Casey
Cover printed by Art Print, Taylor, Pa.
Book printed and bound by Maple Press, York, Pa.
Date printed: April 2011
Printed in the United States of America

10 9 8 7 6 5 4 3 2 1

This book is printed on acid-free paper.

CONTENTS

LIST OF ILLUSTRATIONS AND TABLES

PREFACE

The Truth About series—updated and expanded to include 20 volumes—seeks to identify the most pressing health issues and social challenges confronting our nation's youth. Adolescence is the period between the onset of puberty and the attainment of adult roles and responsibilities. Adolescence is also a time of storm, stress, and risk-taking for many young people. During adolescence, a person's health is influenced by biological, psychological, and social factors, all of which interact with one's environment—family, peers, school, and community. It is a time when teenagers experience profound changes.

With the latest available statistics and new insights that have emerged from ongoing research, the Truth About series seeks to help young people build a foundation of information as they face some of the challenges that will affect their health and well-being. These challenges include high-risk behaviors, such as alcohol, tobacco, and other drug use; sexual behaviors that can lead to adolescent pregnancy and sexually transmitted diseases (STDs), such as HIV/AIDS; mental health concerns, such as depression and suicide; learning disorders and disabilities, which are often associated with school failures and school drop-outs; serious family problems, including domestic violence and abuse; and lifestyle factors, which increase adolescents' risk for noncommunicable diseases, such as diabetes and cardiovascular disease, among others.

Broader underlying factors also influence adolescent health. These include socioeconomic circumstances, such as poverty, available health care, and the political and social situations in which young people live. Although these factors can negatively affect adolescent health and well-being, as well as school performance, many of these negative health outcomes are preventable with the proper knowledge and information.

With prevention in mind, the writers and editors of each topical volume in the Truth About series have tried to provide cutting-edge information that is supported by research and scientific evidence. Vital facts are presented that inform youth about the challenges experienced during adolescence, while special features seek to dispel common myths and misconceptions. Some of the main topics explored include abuse, alcohol, death and dying, divorce, drugs, eating disorders, family life, fear and depression, rape, sexual behavior and unplanned pregnancy, smoking, and violence. All volumes discuss risk-taking behaviors and their consequences, healthy choices, prevention, available treatments, and where to get help.

In this new edition of the series, we also have added eight new titles in areas of increasing significance to today's youth. ADHD, or attention-deficit/hyperactivity disorder, and learning disorders are diagnosed with increasing frequency, and many students have observed or know of classmates receiving treatment for these conditions, even if they have not themselves received this diagnosis. Gambling is gaining currency in our culture, as casinos open and expand in many parts of the country, and the Internet offers easy access for this addictive behavior. Another consequence of our increasingly "online" society, unfortunately, is the presence of online predators. Environmental hazards represent yet another danger, and it is important to provide unbiased information about this topic to our youth. Suicide, which for many years has been a "silent epidemic," is now gaining recognition as a major public health problem throughout the life span, including the teenage and young adult years. We now also offer an overview of illness and disease in a volume that includes the major conditions of particular interest and concern to youth. In addition to illness, however, it is essential to emphasize health and its promotion, and this is especially apparent in the volumes on physical fitness and stress management.

It is our intent that each book serve as an accessible, authoritative resource that young people can turn for accurate and meaningful answers to their specific questions. The series can help them research particular problems and provide an up-to-date evidence base. It is also designed with parents, teachers, and counselors in mind so that they have a reliable resource that they can share with youth who seek their guidance.

Finally, we have tried to provide unbiased facts rather than subjective opinions. Our goal is to help elevate the health of the public with an emphasis on its most precious component—our youth. As young people face the challenges of an increasingly complex world, we as educators want them to be armed with the most powerful weapon available—knowledge.

Robert N. Golden, M.D.
Fred L. Peterson, Ph.D.
General Editors

HOW TO
USE THIS BOOK

NOTE TO STUDENTS

Knowledge is power. By possessing knowledge you have the ability to make decisions, ask follow-up questions, or know where to go to obtain more information. In the world of health, that is power! That is the purpose of this book—to provide you the power you need to obtain unbiased, accurate information and *The Truth About Family Life.*

Topics in each volume of The Truth About series are arranged in alphabetical order, from A to Z. Each of these entries defines its topic and explains in detail the particular issue. At the end of most entries are cross-references to related topics. A list of all topics by letter can be found in the table of contents or at the back of the book in the index.

How have these books been compiled? First, the publisher worked with me to identify some of the country's leading authorities on key issues in health education. These individuals were asked to identify some of the major concerns that young people have about such topics. The writers read the literature, spoke with health experts, and incorporated their own life and professional experiences to pull together the most up-to-date information on health issues, particularly those of interest to adolescents and of concern in *Healthy People 2010.*

Throughout the alphabetical entries, the reader will find sidebars that separate Fact from Fiction. There are Question-and-Answer boxes that attempt to address the most common questions that youths ask about sensitive topics. In addition, readers will find a special feature called "Teens Speak"—case studies of teens with personal stories related to the topic in hand.

This may be one of the most important books you will ever read. Please share it with your friends, families, teachers, and classmates. Remember, you possess the power to control your future. One way to affect your course is through the acquisition of knowledge. Good luck and keep healthy.

NOTE TO LIBRARIANS

This book, along with the rest of The Truth About series, serves as a wonderful resource for young researchers. It contains a variety of facts, case studies, and further readings that the reader can use to help answer questions, formulate new questions, or determine where to go to find more information. Even though the topics may be considered delicate by some, don't be afraid to ask patrons if they have questions. Feel free to direct them to the appropriate sources, but do not press them if you encounter reluctance. The best we can do as educators is to let young people know that we are there when they need us.

Mark J. Kittleson, Ph.D.
Adviser to the First Edition

FAMILY LIFE IN AMERICA

Although families exist in every society, their organization, cultural role, and responsibilities can vary greatly from place to place. Despite these variations, in almost every society, the family has six basic social functions:

- Regulating sexual behavior by limiting whom people may marry, when, and under what conditions
- Assuming responsibility for reproduction
- Nurturing and protecting children and providing emotional support for adults
- Teaching children and other new members of a society what they need to know in order to participate in that society
- Producing and consuming goods. In some societies, the family is the center of economic production and its members produce most of what they consume. In other societies, including American society, families produce little of what they consume.
- Determining an individual's ascribed status in society— that is, his or her status at birth. The status of children in almost every society, and therefore their life chances, are based on their parents' race, ethnicity, wealth, and related social factors

NEW IN THE REVISED EDITION

In the United States, the number of family households was expected to reach 78 million in 2010, up from 68 million households in 1975.

1

Although each household is unique in some way, the sheer number suggests that the family experience will grow more diverse as the population grows. Family life has already evolved significantly: By 2010, the number of families headed by a married couple has fallen to 52 percent, the lowest number in American history.

In this new edition of *The Truth About Family Life,* you will find updated information on family life in the modern United States, complete with its challenges. New articles have been added to expand discussions of such issues as privacy and family boundaries; young family members' desire for more independence; the role of family counseling; how puberty and sexual development can play a role in family dynamics; the ways in which families communicate; the role of ethnicity in society's expectations; and information about the growing study of birth order and how it can play a role in a person's development and success.

HISTORY OF THE FAMILY IN AMERICA

In the 1950s, according to comparison data in the U.S. census report of 2001, about two-thirds of children in the United States lived in families that consisted of a mother, father, and their children. In most of these families, the father was the breadwinner and the mother cared for the home and children. By 2002, only 10 percent of families fit this portrait of the traditional family. The traditional family has become just one of many family forms.

According to family demographer Jay D. Teachman, changing economic patterns was one reason for the shift in family life. The 1950s were a time of economic affluence for many families. Government-backed programs provided inexpensive home loans, support for veterans to attend college, and other benefits. The minimum wage was high enough to support a family of three above the poverty level.

By the 1960s and 1970s, families were finding it harder and harder to survive on the income of one wage earner. To maintain their standard of living, many families needed more than one wage earner. Many wives and mothers returned to the labor force to help their family make ends meet. The women's movement of the 1960s encouraged this trend. By 2008, 71 percent of married women worked outside the home, according to the Bureau of Labor Statistics.

Teachman and other researchers observed that as women achieved greater economic independence, they were less likely to stay in unhappy marriages. The rate of divorce—the legal ending of a marriage—increased dramatically during the last 40 years of the 20th century. Data from the National Center for Health Statistics (NCHA) show that the divorce rate nearly doubled between 1960 and 1970. It continued to climb until 1978, when it reached a high of 23 per 1,000 married women. It dropped slightly to about 20 per 1,000 during the 1980s and leveled off during the 1990s. By 2005, the divorce rate was 3.6 per 1,000 people. This was the lowest rate since 1970.

The increasing participation of women in the labor force also affected the way families interacted. For many couples, a more equal division of financial responsibilities led to greater equality in the division of household labor and child care responsibilities.

THE NEW FAMILY

If Americans are not living in nuclear families headed by two parents, what kind of families are they living in? More people today are choosing to marry later. Census Bureau data show that the percentage of married-couple households dropped from more than three out of every four households in 1950 (78 percent) to slightly more than one-half (52 percent) in 2000. However, in 2009, this number increased to 73 percent. The percentage of households occupied by one person increased from 11 percent in 1950 to 29 percent in 2008.

In 1959, nearly half of all women were under the age of 19 when they married. Since the mid-1950s, the median age at first marriage has been rising steadily, with the largest increases occurring since 1980. By 2008, the median age at first marriage had reached 28.1 years for men and 25.9 years for women. In 2008, according to the Census Bureau, the ratio of men who never married by age 45 was 12 percent higher than that for women. Of those people who never married, 34.6 percent were men and 28.1 percent were women.

Because of the high divorce rate, many children are likely to be reared in a home that does not include their two biological parents. In 1972, 73 percent of children lived with their married biological parents; by 2009, less than one-third of all children lived in this type of family.

Between 1970 and 2009, the number of single-parent families tripled from 4 million to almost 20 million. In 2008, the Census Bureau found that 21.1 percent of U.S. households included married-couple families with their own children.

Blended and reblended families are created when a divorced or widowed parent marries a new spouse. These families are becoming more common as divorced parents remarry, half of them more than once. In 1998, the last year in which the Census Bureau collected data on remarriages, in 46 percent of new marriages, the husband, wife, or both had been previously married.

Census Bureau researchers predict that more than one-third of all children in the United States will live in a blended family before they reach the age of 18. Census 2004 data show that in 2004, an estimated 5.8 million children were living with a stepparent.

Americans are having fewer children. In 1900, married women had, on average, five children. Other data from the NCHS show wide fluctuations in the **fertility rate**—the average number of children a woman has in her lifetime. In the late 1950s, the average woman gave birth to 3.5 children during her lifetime. The fertility rate dropped to a low of 1.8 births per woman in 1972, then climbed slightly and stayed at between 2.0 and 2.1 births per woman from the early 1990s through 2003. In 2007, NCHS data showed the fertility rate was 69.5 births per 1,000 women aged 15–44 years.

Between 1960 and 1990, the declining fertility rate led to smaller families. During this time period, the average number of persons per family decreased from 3.67 to 3.18. Census Bureau data show in 2009 that in married-couple households the average number of persons living in the family was 3.25. Overall, 2009 households included an average of 2.61 individuals. The proportion of married couples with children also has declined, according to the Census Bureau. In 2003, only 23 percent of households in the United States included married couples with children, a dramatic decrease from 40 percent in 1970. In 2008 this number decreased further to 31.0 percent.

The percentage of unmarried women who gave birth to children climbed from 5 percent in 1960 to 39.7 percent in 2006, according to data from the National Center for Health Statistics. Teens accounted for 34 percent of all births to unmarried women in 2002, a decrease from 50 percent in 1970. The decrease was due to the fact that a greater number of older unmarried women were choosing to become mothers. The total number of births to unmarried mothers increased 20 percent between 2002 and 2006.

Many of the women counted as unmarried mothers by the Census Bureau are living with a partner. The practice of living together without marriage is known as **cohabitation**. According to data from the census, 5.4 million couples were cohabitating in 2008. About 60 percent of those couples were between 25 and 44 years old, and more than one-third (36 percent) had children under the age of 15. More than half of heterosexual couples who planned to marry lived together before they were wed. In 1965, that figure was 10 percent. Other couples choose cohabitation because they wish to share their lives with a partner and have children even though they do not wish to marry.

Of these cohabitating couples, 4.9 million lived with someone of the opposite sex and just under 674,000 had same-sex partners. Many of these same-sex partners have not married because they are not allowed to marry. Although same-sex couples can marry in Massachusetts, other states forbid marriages between partners of the same sex. Some cities and businesses recognize same-sex couples as domestic partners.

Of the same-sex couples who have children, these families are formed by previous heterosexual relationships, from the process of adoption, or through medical procedures such as **artificial insemination,** the injection of a man's sperm into a woman's vagina using a syringe. Researchers from the National Adoption Information Clearinghouse estimate that between 2 and 6 million same-sex couples in the United States are rearing between 6 and 14 million children.

Some of these couples are choosing to build families through adoption. About 100,000 children are adopted each year in the United States. In 2004, 1.6 million children under age 18 were living with adoptive parents. In 2002, about 20 percent of all adoptions involved children from countries outside the United States. Data from 2003 show international adoptions increased by 7.23 percent between 2002 and 2003. However, in 2008, the U.S. State Department reported a decrease in international adoptions between 2004 and 2008. Open adoption, in which communication occurs between the birth and adoptive parents and child, is becoming more common.

Another important influence on family life has been the increasing number of elderly people in the United States. The 2008 census revealed that 12.8 percent of the population—39 million people in all—were age 65 or older. These people are spending a greater percentage of their lives without young children in their households. However, as people age, they are more likely to require health care and assistance with daily living. When an elderly parent is no longer able to care for himself or herself, family members may be called upon to provide support.

As family structures evolve in response to social, economic, and technological influences, the ways in which Americans think about family life are changing. It is likely that the "new" American family will continue to change even more during the 21st century. Learning about the diverse family structures in which families live can help you to find creative and flexible options for raising children, maintaining intimate relationships, and finding fulfillment.

RISKY BUSINESS SELF-TEST

Everyone has experienced some sort of family. So you could say that you are, indeed, an expert on families. But how much do you really know about building healthy families and relationships?

To test your knowledge about families and relationships, grab a pencil and separate piece of paper and jot down your answers to this multiple-choice quiz. Following the self-test are the answers and explanations to rate your score.

What's my family and relationship IQ?

1. If my parent hits me in anger,

    a. I deserve it. It's just normal discipline.

    b. I hit him or her back.

    c. I seek help.

2. If my partner hits me,

    a. I put up with it because he or she apologizes later.

    b. I leave and seek help.

    c. I take it as a sign of how much he or she loves me.

3. If I become a teen parent,

    a. I will probably finish high school and go on to college.

    b. I will probably marry my child's other parent.

    c. I will probably remain single, need to take a part-time job to pay for my child's expenses, and need a lot of support to finish high school.

4. The best way to handle an argument with my parents is to

    a. run to my room and lock the door.

    b. talk to my friends about it.

    c. wait until I've calmed down then talk to them about my feelings.

5. If I marry and eventually divorce,

    a. I will never be able to face my family and friends again.

    b. I will remain single for the rest of my life.

    c. I will probably have a rough time for a while, but I'll survive and learn from the experience and probably marry again.

6. If I marry while I'm in my teens,

    a. I decrease the chance that I will divorce.

    b. I increase the chance that I will divorce.

    c. I won't affect the chance that I will divorce.

7. If my parents divorce, but I get along well with each of them and they don't draw me into their arguments, it's most likely that

    a. I'll experience behavioral and emotional problems and have difficulty forming intimate relationships as an adult.

    b. I'll be just as emotionally healthy as kids whose parents aren't divorced.

    c. I'll be the only kid in my school with divorced parents.

8. Intimate relationships between two people of the same sex are

    a. markedly different from other intimate relationships.

    b. similar to relationships between heterosexual couples.

    c. unhealthy for children to grow up in.

9. Single parents

    a. provide their children with the care they need.

    b. can't provide healthy homes for their children.

    c. are always poor.

10. If my parents divorce and remarry,

    a. I'll be disloyal to my biological parent if I become close to my stepparent.

    b. it will probably be difficult, but I can handle it.

    c. I'll be angry at my parents for divorcing and remarrying.

Answer key

1. c. Any act of violence from one family member to another is cause for concern. If your parent strikes you, find a safe place, such as a friend's home, and arrange to talk to your parent with a counselor or friend. If any parent strikes you repeatedly, seek out a domestic violence shelter and get regular help from a counselor, teacher, pastor, friend's parent, or other adult.

2. b. If your partner hits, slaps, or otherwise physically assaults you, he or she is abusing you. Leave. Seek help from someone you trust, such as a teacher, pastor, parent, friend's parent, doctor, or other adult.

3. c. Even though most teen mothers believe they will marry their child's father, the reality is that less than 8 percent will do so within one year. In fact, according to the Alan Guttmacher Institute, a nonprofit organization that performs research on reproduction and health, less than 40 percent of mothers who have a child before age 18 ever complete high school, and fewer teen fathers complete high school than those who wait to become parents until they are 21 years old. Their low educational levels make it unlikely that they will ever qualify for a job that pays well.

4. c. Tightly knit families discuss important things instead of avoiding them. Often the best way to resolve a dispute, or at least to learn to live with it, is to allow each family member to clearly describe his or her position in a safe environment such as a family meeting with established rules.

5. c. Divorce is usually accompanied by emotional pain, sadness, anger, and many other difficult feelings. But when people choose to divorce, it's usually because they are not satisfied with their current relationship and they believe they can create a better one with someone else. Both children and adults experience divorce in a series of stages similar to those described by Elisabeth Kübler-Ross in her book *On Death and Dying* for terminally ill patients: denial, anger,

bargaining, depression and acceptance. About two-thirds of people who divorce each year eventually remarry.

6. b. One of the most important predictors of divorce is age at first marriage. Teenage marriages are the most likely to end in divorce, probably because teens are still in the midst of developing their own value systems, identities, and choosing careers. One-third of marriages that occur before the woman is 18 end in divorce within three years. Half of those marriages end within 10 years.

7. b. Several studies have linked parental divorce to behavioral problems in children. However, the conflict that often surrounds divorce, not the divorce itself, appears to be the trigger for behavioral problems in children of divorced parents. Current research shows that parental conflict is a greater threat to children's well-being than is family structure.

8. b. Researchers have found few differences between heterosexual and homosexual couples except the sex of the partner. Same-sex couples fall in love, feel the same passions, experience the same doubts, and feel the same commitments that heterosexual couples do.

9. a. Single parents face many challenges, including reduced income, lack of family time, and the lack of another adult to share parenting and household responsibilities with. However, a single-parent family can provide a healthy environment for its members. Most single parents give their children the structure, values, and nurturance that they need. Children thrive in a warm, supportive home, regardless of whether it is headed by one or two parents. Children adjust better when they have a good relationship with a single parent than when they live with two parents who are in constant conflict.

10. b. The adjustment to a stepparent is often difficult for children of all ages, especially young teens. A stepparent is not a replacement parent, and developing a relationship with a stepparent does not mean you're abandoning your biological parent. There's no rule that says you can't love two adults who play parental roles in your life. In fact, most teens are pleased when their custodial parent remarries. One reason may be that money problems tend to decrease with remarriage. In one study, the most frequently used word used by teens to describe their reactions to their custodial parent's remarriage was *happy; satisfied* and *pleased* were the second and third most common terms.

See the Hotline and Help Sites section of this book for several places to contact if you want to talk with someone about a stressful family situation and what you can do to begin to feel better.

See also: Arguments and the Family; Divorce and Families; Families, Divided; Gay Parents; Marriage and Family, Changes in; Single-Parent Families; Stepparents; Teenage Parents; Teens in Trouble; Violence and the Family

A-TO-Z ENTRIES

■ ADOPTION

Adoption is the legal transfer of the biological parents' rights to a child to another adult or couple. The adoptive parent or parents assume all of the parental rights and responsibilities of the biological parents, including care and supervision of the child, nurture, training, education, physical and emotional health, and financial support.

RATES IN THE UNITED STATES AND ABROAD

In 2008, 1.6 million children under the age of 18 were living with adults who had assumed legal responsibility for them. These adults are known as the child's **adoptive parents**. About 2 percent of all children in the United States are adopted. An additional 473,000 children above the age of 18 were living with adoptive parents. These 2.1 million adopted children represent 2.5 percent of all children in U.S. households.

The 2000 census data concerning adoptions is incomplete. Census takers did not ask whether adopted children were biologically related to their adoptive parents. For example, some adults adopt nieces or nephews. Others adopt stepchildren. The census data also does not indicate whether a child was adopted through a government agency or private organization.

Information related to those issues is available from public agencies and private organizations that place children in adoptive homes. According to the National Council for Adoption (NCFA), for instance, more than 5 million adults and children in the United States have been adopted. The group estimates that more than 100,000 children are adopted each year. In 2005, 51,000 children were adopted with public agency involvement.

Other data collected by the NCFA shows that slightly more than half (50.9 percent) of those who adopt a child are related to that child in some way. Often, these adoptions simply formalize an existing arrangement. Most related adoptions involve a stepparent (usually a stepfather) adopting his wife's children. Many states have a streamlined process for stepparent adoptions. However, in some states, parents must be married for at least one year before such an adoption will be approved.

Unrelated adoptions account for slightly less than half of all adoptions. Almost 40 percent of unrelated adoptions in the United States are handled by government agencies, usually a state social-services

Education Level of Adoptive Parents of Special-Needs Children

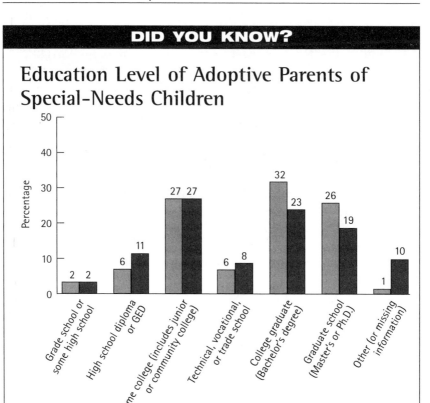

According to the U.S. Census Bureau in 2000, adoptive parents were much more likely than biological parents or stepparents to have college degrees. That trend continues. In a four-year study of 270 successful adoptive parents who adopted children, in this case with special needs, researchers at the University of Texas at Austin found that more than half of the adoptive parents whom they surveyed had completed either a bachelor's or graduate degree.

Source: *A Report to Congress on Barriers and Success Factors in Adoptions from Foster Care: Perspectives of Families and Staff Supported by the Adoption Opportunities Program*, U.S. Department of Health and Human Services, Administration for Children & Families, 2007.

agency. The National Council for Adoption reports that in 1992, about one-third (29 percent) of unrelated adoptions were handled by private agencies. This rate has continued to hold steady. Some adoptions are privately arranged. A pregnant woman or her attorney may reach an agreement with an individual or couple eager to adopt her unborn child. Such adoptions make up the other 31 percent of unrelated adoptions. More recently, intercountry adoptions comprised a greater percentage of all unrelated adoptions (21.7 percent in 2002).

State laws govern the adoption of children in the United States. While all states require that adoptive parents be at least 21 years of age, age requirements vary from state to state. Americans who wish to adopt a child from another country must be U.S. citizens and at least 25 years of age. Adoptive parents may be married or single. They may already have children or they may be childless.

Healthy, white infants are the most likely to be adopted. The National Adoption Information Clearinghouse (NAIC) estimates that there are 127,000 domestic and international adoptions each year. However, according to the NAIC, adoption is less likely for children who are eight years or older, have siblings, belong to a racial or ethnic minority group, or have mental, emotional, or physical disabilities. In 1997, Congress passed the Adoption and Safe Families Act (ASFA). The law was designed to promote the adoption of children who face barriers in finding adoptive homes. For the purposes of adoption, the ASFA classified children who face one or more of these barriers as "children with special needs." State agencies provide financial and other support to parents who adopt children with special needs as defined by the ASFA.

Many children with special needs are in the care of public agencies. Children who have been abused, neglected, or abandoned by their birth parents are placed in state foster care. These children live with **foster parents** who care for them while their birth parents receive counseling and other services. Foster care programs are designed to help birth parents reunite with their children. However, if reuniting is not possible, the agency may take away, or terminate, the birth parents' rights to the child. The ASFA requires courts to seek termination of parental rights for children who have been in foster care for 15 out of the previous 22 months, except in special circumstances.

The National Council for Adoption estimates that the ASFA has led to 11,000 additional adoptions each year. The number of children adopted from foster care rose from 31,000 in 1997 to 50,000 in 2001, according to the Adoption and Foster Care Analysis and Reporting System (AFCARS). Of the 263,000 children in foster care, 18 percent were adopted. Most of the others who left foster care were reunited with their birth parents, living with other relatives, or were **emancipated,** meaning they were older than 16 years of age and able to live on their own as adults.

Many children in foster care are waiting to be adopted. About three-fourths (76 percent) of those children have been in foster care for three years or longer. Their average age is 10 years. Thirty-seven percent are African American, 12 percent are Hispanic, and 34 percent are white. Only 25,000 children in foster care in 2001 according to AFCARS were living with foster parents who planned to adopt them.

In 2008, the U.S. State Department reported that there were 17,438 international adoptions. This number represents a decrease in international adoptions over the past four years. However, adoptions from Africa have increased from 9 percent in 2007 to 13 percent in 2008, representing 2,315 adopted children. Other country adoption statistics include Asia with 6,735 children, or 39 percent; and 3,074 children from Europe, or 18 percent; North American adoptions included 4,630 children, or 27 percent; and 439 adoptions took place from South America, representing 3 percent of all international adoptions.

TRANSRACIAL ADOPTION

A transracial adoption is the adoption of children whose racial or ethnic backgrounds differ from those of their adoptive parents. In the United States, most transracial adoptions involve white parents and children of another race. Transracial adoption rates appear to be increasing. In 1987, estimates from the National Health Interview Survey (NHIS) indicated that about 8 percent of adoptions involved parents and children of different races. The data provided by the 2000 Census found that more than 17 percent of adopted children were of a different race than the head of the family.

The law that governs transracial adoption is the Howard M. Metzenbaum Multiethnic Placement Act of 1994 (MEPA). MEPA prohibits any organization involved in adoptive or foster care placement that receives federal assistance from delaying or denying the placement of a child on the basis of the race, color, or national origin of the child or the adoptive or foster parent. In 1996, MEPA was amended by the Interethnic Adoption Provisions Law, which forbids agencies from denying or delaying placement of a child for adoption solely on the basis of race or national origin. The 1978 Indian Child Welfare Act strictly limits the adoption of Native American children by adults who are not Native American. The act requires that agencies begin by trying to place the child with a member of his or her extended family. If that is not possible, agencies should try to place the child with other members of his or her tribe. If agencies are unable to do so, the child may be placed with a Native American family that is not a member of the child's tribe.

Despite the increase in the number of transracial adoptions in the United States over the last 20 years, sociologists, child development experts, and others involved with adoption continue to debate the effects of placing a child in a family with a different racial or ethnic background. The debate began in earnest in 1972, when the National Association of Black Social Workers (NABSW) published a position paper "vehemently" opposing the placement of African-American children with white families. The NABSW called for African-American children to be placed only with African-American families, whether in foster care or for adoption, and argued that "black children belong, physically, psychologically and culturally, in black families in order that they receive the total sense of themselves and develop a sound projection of their future."

The NABSW reaffirmed its opposition to transracial adoption in both 1977 and 1985. In 1985, the president of the NABSW testified before the Senate Committee on Labor and Human Resources. His testimony focused on two main points. The first was that African-American children who grow up in white families suffer severe identity problems because they are not fully accepted by white communities and do not have significant ties with other African Americans. The second was that transracially adopted African-American children do not develop coping mechanisms necessary to function in a society that is inherently racist. In 1994, the NABSW expanded their position to emphasize that children of African ancestry should be placed in the care of relatives or adopted by African-American families. The NABSW emphasized that transracial adoption of African-American children should take place only after efforts for same-race adoption placement have been exhausted.

A growing body of research does not support either argument. It suggests that most children who are adopted across races or cultures fare well. Rita Simon, a professor in the School of Public Affairs at the Washington College of Law at American University, and Howard Alstein, a professor in the School of Social Work at the University of Maryland, conducted one of the most comprehensive studies of transracial adoption. The longitudinal study, which began in 1972, followed 206 families with 218 children, including birth and adopted children. In 1990, the researchers contacted 98 of the children who had participated in the 1972 study. Based on their interviews with the children as adolescents and adults, Simon and Alstein concluded that the transracially adopted children were comfortable with their racial identity. However, as adults, 91 percent of the transracially adopted children said parents who adopt a child from another culture or race need to be sensitive to racial issues. Nine percent said they should reconsider their decision to adopt a child of another race.

In 1983, Arnold R. Silverman, a professor of sociology at Nassau Community College in New York, reviewed nearly a dozen studies of transracial adoption. His analysis showed that about 75 percent of transracially adopted preadolescents and younger children adjust well to their adoptive families. Ten years later, Silverman published "Outcomes of Transracial Adoption," in which he again reviewed existing research on the adjustment of transracially adopted children. Based on this second review, he concluded that transracial adoption is a viable means of providing stable homes for nonwhite children awaiting placement.

GAY PARENTS AND ADOPTION

By law, same-sex couples are allowed to adopt children in 23 states and the District of Columbia. However, county judges within each state may prohibit adoption within their jurisdictions. In 2010, an appeals court in Florida ruled that the state's ban on gays adopting children was unconstitutional and overturned it. Prior to this ruling, Florida was the only state that still had a ban on same-sex adoption without exception. Although most other states do not legally prohibit same-sex couples from adopting children, they discourage all single people (not married) from adopting children, including gays. As of 2010, only Massachusetts, Connecticut, New Hampshire, Vermont, Iowa, and the District of Columbia recognize same-sex marriage as legal.

In most cases, when a child is born to or adopted by a same-sex couple, only one parent is legally recognized as the parent. For instance, if a same-sex couple chooses to have a child through **artificial insemination,** only the birth mother has parental rights. The other partner does not have any parental rights—including the right to make decisions about the child's medical care—or responsibilities—including the responsibility to pay child support if the couple separates—unless he or she formally adopts the child. The American Association of Pediatrics (AAP) argues that "children deserve to know that their relationships with both of their parents are stable and legally recognized," whether their parents are of the same or different sexes. Thus, the AAP supports the adoption of children by the second parent in families headed by a couple of the same sex. The AAP bases its recommendations on "a considerable body of professional literature" that shows that children who grow up in one- or two-parent gay or lesbian households "can have the same advantages and the same expectations for health, adjustment and development as can children whose parents are heterosexual."

In 2003, researchers from the Evan B. Donalds Adoption Institute published *Adoption by Lesbians and Gays: A National Survey of Adoption Agency Policies, Practices, and Attitudes*. The study, which was conducted between 1999 and 2000, surveyed adoption agencies as to whether they permitted adoption of children by gays and lesbians and how many children they actually placed with same-sex parents. The study also examined the attitudes of birth parents and agencies regarding the adoption of children by gays and lesbians.

Survey results show that as lesbians and gays are adopting children from both public and private agencies at a growing rate, the practice is becoming more acceptable. Adoption program directors from 277 private agencies and 30 public agencies responded to the survey. About 60 percent accepted adoption applications from gays and lesbians. About 39 percent had placed at least one child with gay and lesbian parents between 1999 and 2000. Of the 91,118 adoption placements reported by the agencies, 1,206 (1.3 percent) were with gays and lesbians. Researchers caution that this number may be considerably less than the actual current placements because most agencies do not keep records of the sexual orientation of adoptive parents. Of the agencies that responded to the survey, 25 percent said prospective birth parents did not want to place their child with gays or lesbians. On the other hand, 15 percent of all agencies said birth parents had requested or chosen lesbian or gay prospective adoptive parents for their child. Researchers also asked whether agency staff would be interested in receiving training to work more effectively with prospective gay and lesbian adoptive parents. Almost half (48 percent) of agencies indicated they would be interested in receiving such training.

Fact Or Fiction?

Open adoption causes problems for adopted children.

The Facts: Adoptions occur along a spectrum of openness, ranging from direct contact and communication among all parties to complete confidentiality. Open adoption, in which interactions take place between birth and adoptive parents—and often the adopted child—are becoming more common. While open adoption may not be the best situation for every adopted child, a growing body of research shows that open adoption may actually be good not only for the adopted child, but also for the child's adoptive and birth parents. Findings from the Minnesota/Texas Adoption Research Project, a study that compared open adoption to other types of adoption, debunk many myths about open adoption. Results from the study showed that open adoption does not

- Prompt birth mothers to try to "reclaim" their children
- Make it harder for birth mothers to resolve grief. In fact, birth mothers in open adoption situations show better grief resolution than those in confidential adoptions
- Make adoptive parents feel less in control. Adoptive parents have a greater sense of permanence about their relationship with their adopted child
- Cause children to feel confused about who their parents are, the roles of their birth parents versus their adoptive parents
- Appear to negatively influence children's self-esteem.

FAMILY DYNAMICS

The introduction of a new child into a family changes the way the family functions and how members interact. While related adoptions may not substantially change a child's daily routine, unrelated adoptions almost always involve a significant change in a child's life. That change usually includes the establishment of new relationships. Early results from a study at the University of Minnesota's Center for Twin and Family Research, Sibling Interaction and Behavior Study (SIBS) may shed some light on the effects of introducing an adopted child into a family. The SIBS study, which began in 1999, examines how siblings interact and influence one another and how family dynamics can affect the psychological health of teens. (In 2010, the SIBS was conducting a second follow-up study.) To determine psychological health, researchers measured negative behaviors such as delinquency, antisocial attitudes, aggression, substance abuse, and other problem behaviors. They also measured positive characteristics such as sense of well-being, a positive self-identity, and academic achievement.

Q & A

Question: How can I explain that my adopted sister is my "real" sister?

Answer: There are many ways to build a family. An adoptive family is as real a family as one in which parents and children are biologically related. You can start by encouraging your friends, parents, and teachers to use correct terminology. The language people use reflects and influences their beliefs, and the language that people use about adoption sometimes suggests that adoptive families are somehow inferior to biologically related families. Tell your friends that your sister is your real sister even though you do not share the same birth parents. She is a member of your family.

Of the 600 families in the SIBS study, 400 include an adopted child. Early findings from the study, published in 2002, showed little difference in psychological functioning between children reared in adoptive families and those reared in **birth families**. Sibling relationships appeared to be equally close and loving among adopted and biological siblings. While adopted children and parents reported more conflict, they also said they felt as attached to one another as children and parents in birth families.

Adoptive siblings in the study do not share genetically linked personality traits such as shyness or gregariousness. They do, however, show remarkable similarity in academic achievement. According to SIBS researchers, this finding suggests that parental influence plays a major role in academic success. In contrast, younger siblings were more likely to display problem behaviors such as smoking, drinking, or disobedience when older siblings engaged in such behaviors. Preliminary results from the SIBS study suggest that sibling influence may be a more important determinant of problem behavior than parental influence.

Until the 1970s, adoption was rarely discussed and often kept a secret from the children who were adopted. Few adopted children ever met their birth parents and birth parents rarely met adoptive parents. Today, these confidential adoptions, in which the adoptive family and birth parents do not communicate, fall at one end of a spectrum of adoption practices. In the middle of the spectrum is semi-open adoption, in which birth and adoptive families communicate through a third party, such as an agency caseworker or attorney. At the other end of the spectrum, and becoming more common, is open adoption. In open adoptions, the birth and adoptive parents and the child communicate directly with one another. Interactions may range from letters, e-mails, and telephone calls to visits based on the needs and interests of the members of both families.

According to the National Adoption Information Clearinghouse (NAIC), adoptive parents who choose open adoption try to minimize the child's loss of relationships and acknowledge all connections in the child's life. A growing body of research supports the view that openness in adoption can be a positive experience for both children and parents. Findings from the Minnesota/Texas Adoption Research Project, a longitudinal study that compares open adoption with other types of adoption, suggests that ongoing contact between birth parents and adopted children increases satisfaction with the adoption. Of the 190 families in the study, 46 were in direct or indirect contact with each other since the child was placed with an adoptive family. Most respondents who had ongoing contact reported that they were either satisfied or very satisfied with the level of openness shown by the child's birth mother: 83.7 percent of the adopted adolescents, 93.5 percent of the adoptive mothers, and 84.8 percent of the adoptive fathers. The teens reported that they hoped their contact with their birth mother stayed the same (55.8 percent) or increased (41.9 percent) in the future. Only one adolescent (2.3 percent) hoped for a decrease.

When the researchers compared the teens who were in contact with their birth mothers to those who were not, they found that adolescents who had contact with their birth mothers reported higher degrees of satisfaction with the level of adoption openness and with the intensity of their contact with their birth mother than did adolescents who had no contact. Teens were least satisfied with openness about adoption during middle adolescence (ages 14–16), slightly more satisfied during early or late adolescence.

In a 2008 study published in the *British Journal of Social Work,* the authors found that the issue of adoption relationships is complex overall; generally, however, the experience is a positive one and should be encouraged for anyone who seeks that option.

In summary, about 100,000 children are adopted each year in the United States, and in 2004, 1.6 million children under age 18 were living with adoptive parents, half of which were related adoptions, usually involving a stepparent adopting a new spouse's child. The Adoption and Safe Families Act (ASFA) of 1997 was designed to increase adoption of children who are eight years or older, members of a minority group, in a group of siblings, or who have mental, emotional, or physical disabilities.

Children who have been abused, neglected, or abandoned by their birth parents are placed in a state foster care system, in which children live with foster parents who care for them while their birth parents receive counseling and other services. If the children cannot be safely reunited with their parents, they become eligible for adoption.

Controversy still surrounds the practice of transracial adoption, in which parents adopt children of different racial or ethnic backgrounds. Some researchers argue that transracial adoption is a means of providing safe, permanent homes to the many minority children who are in foster care and awaiting adoption. Others hold that minority children experience problems with racial identification when they are reared in white families. Although controversy also surrounds the rights of same-sex couples to adopt children, studies show that children who grow up in one- or two-parent gay or lesbian households do as well emotionally and socially as children with heterosexual parents. Open adoption, in which communication occurs between the birth and adoptive parents and child, is becoming more common.

See also: Divorce and Families; Families, Blended; Families, Racially Mixed; Family, The New; Gay Parents; Marriage and Family, Changes in; Stepparents

FURTHER READING
Eldridge, Sherrie. *Forever Fingerprints: An Amazing Discovery for Adopted Children.* Warren, N.J.: EMK Publishing, 2007.

Keck, Gregory C. *Parenting Adopted Adolescents: Understanding and Appreciating Their Journeys*. Colorado Springs, Colo.: NavPress, 2009.

Slade, Suzanne B. *Adopted: The Ultimate Teen Guide*. It Happened to Me. Lanham, Md.: The Scarecrow Press, Inc., 2007.

■ ARGUMENTS AND THE FAMILY

A certain degree of conflict exists in all families. When conflicts are handled directly and appropriately, they cause few long-term problems. However, when left unresolved, arguments can lead to long-term disagreements and destroy relationships among family members. Families that learn to handle conflict directly can often use conflict to grow closer.

QUARRELS AMONG SIBLINGS

In the United States, most children have at least one **sibling**, a brother or sister. Siblings can be close companions who support and help each other as they grow into adulthood. Most children feel a deeper, stronger affection for their siblings than friends outside the family. Yet many also experience intense competition and resentment of their siblings. Intense sibling rivalries can span a lifetime, starting during early childhood and extending into adulthood. These dual feelings of caring and anger are common in sibling relationships. Those who have such mixed or uncertain feelings are said to be ambivalent.

TEENS SPEAK

Making Peace With My Brother

I can't remember a time when my brother Mike and I didn't fight. We've always had a love-hate relationship, maybe because we're so close in age. He's 17 and I'm 16. When we were younger, we fought about things like which television show to watch or who got to sit in the front seat of the car. Those were little-kid kinds of fights. Eventually we'd make up. Mom or Dad often had to step in, which usually meant that the television got turned off or that both of us had to ride in the backseat.

These days, we fight about politics and ideas. I spend summers working at a garage to make enough money to fix my motorcycle. I barely have a C average at school, except for my art class, where I always get A's. If it weren't for art, I'd probably drop out of school. Mike, on the other hand, is Mr. Successful. He dresses neatly, cuts his hair the same way that our father does, and has a 4.0 grade point average. He'll probably be valedictorian of his class. Last summer, he did an internship at a broker's office.

We've fought for as long as I can remember. I never knew how it affected our parents until the day Mike launched into another lecture about how global warming was just a scare tactic created by environmentalists and I responded by telling him what a selfish pig he was. I didn't know it, but my mom was in the room. When I turned around and saw her crying, I knew that our arguing was hurting our family. I needed to make peace with him. I asked my parents for help. My mom called a counselor, and we went to family therapy sessions for a while. We have weekly family meetings where we've learned to discuss our differences respectfully, without calling each other names or trying to persuade each other that we're right.

Mike and I have agreed to disagree. He'll be leaving for college next year. He's planning to get a degree in business. He told me that one of his goals is to make his first million by the time he's 30. I'm thinking about spending a year or two in the Peace Corps before I go to college. We're still as different as different can be, but we've learned that our differences don't mean we have to be enemies.

Research has shown that conflict among siblings can have positive effects. Arguments with a sibling allow a child to test and develop the skills necessary in resolving conflicts. In a 2009 study published in the journal *Child Development*, research showed that high-quality relationships with siblings were associated with learning how to develop positive conflict processes. However, other researchers have found increases in sibling conflict were linked to increases in symptoms of depression, and increases in sibling intimacy were linked to increases in peer competence for boys and, for girls, decreases in symptoms of depression. In 2007, a 30-year longitudinal study published in the American Psychiatric Association's *Journal of Psychiatry* rated the quality of relationships with siblings and found that poor sibling relationships in childhood may be an important and specific predictor of major depression in adulthood.

According to psychologists Catherine C. Epkins and Angela Dedmon, the research suggests that children's interactions with siblings are affected by birth order and age, gender, and the age difference between the children involved. Older or firstborn children tend to be more aggressive than younger or second-born children. Younger siblings often learn to cajole, negotiate, and compromise; they may become practiced at sensing others' needs and feelings.

The difference in ages among the children in a family may also affect the way that siblings interact. Wyndol Furman, a professor of psychology at the University of Denver, and his colleague Duane Buhrmester, a developmental psychologist at the University of Texas at Dallas, were among the first to examine the effects of age difference on sibling relationships. Their research, supported by a 2010 study published in *Child Development* suggests that siblings who are closer in age tend to experience more conflict and rivalry. Siblings who are farther apart in age tend to argue less and show more affection toward each other. According to this research, three years is the critical age difference: In most of the studies, siblings born one to three years apart were more likely to act aggressively toward each other, while siblings born three or more years apart tended to get along better.

Gender also affects sibling interactions. Although girls are as likely as boys to argue or fight with their siblings, same-sex siblings are more likely to argue than siblings of opposite genders.

As they grow older, children focus on the larger social, psychological, and emotional context of arguments. Instead of being occupied with just the facts, they argue about opinions and ideas including current events, other relationships, and preferences in music, food, or dress. They are better able to discuss their disagreements by clearly expressing their own thoughts and feelings. Older children and teens may use sarcasm, teasing, or insults to show displeasure.

In a 2007 study published in the journal *Child Development*, researchers examined 48 families with children ages five to 10 years old. The findings showed that if parents received training on how to resolve conflict between siblings, then their children learned more positive ways of resolving disputes with siblings. These strategies included negotiations, understanding how blaming has a negative role in conflict resolution, and knowledge of a sibling's view of a situation.

Fact Or Fiction?

Teens fight with their parents about important things.

The Facts: Although conflicts between parents and teens are common and often intense, the things they fight about are not likely to be important. Sociologists such as Brian K. Barber, whose 1994 study of parent-child conflict provided the basis for much current research, reveals that teens and their parents rarely fight openly about economic, religious, social, or political values, or even about sexual activity and drug or alcohol abuse. Conflicts usually focus on more mundane matters, such as helping out around the house. Most of these arguments center on how much freedom teens should have or how soon they should be able to do something (like have the keys to the family car).

A 2010 study published in *Child Development* showed both the rate and overall amount of conflict between parents and teens decreased with age. However, the effect of the conflict increased with age. The increased conflict in early adolescence may be related to the changes that accompany puberty and the need to assert independence. Less stormy relations during late adolescence may occur after parents and teens have successfully renegotiated their relationship.

WHAT WAS IT WE WERE FIGHTING ABOUT?

Conflicts arise in all families and between all members of a family. Some arguments—like who should take out the trash—may be easy to settle. However, when the argument is about a fundamental belief or idea such as religious values or political ideas, it can damage relationships among family members. In most cases, it is not the conflict itself but how it is handled that determines the outcome.

Tightly knit families discuss issues instead of avoiding them. In contrast, when conflict is not handled in a mature and open fashion, it can lead to long-term estrangements between family members.

Often the best way to resolve a dispute, or at least to learn to live with it, is to allow each family member to clearly articulate his or her position. A family conference may provide an environment that allows all family members a chance to state their position in a safe, respectful environment. To set up a family conference, set aside a time and choose a place where everyone can discuss his or her feelings openly. Before the discussion begins, establish ground rules. These may include things such as agreeing that only one person will talk at a time, identifying a signal to indicate that someone would like to speak, agreeing not to interrupt each other, and avoiding name calling. Designate a leader to direct the discussion. Experts recommend that every family conference have a different leader, so that family members change roles. The leader should use open-ended questions like, "How do you feel about what's going on?"

A family conference is not a forum to try to convince anyone that he or she is in the wrong or for parents to educate children about their beliefs. It is a time and place where everyone in the family can express ideas and opinions in a safe environment. The goal is to leave the conference aware of each others' feelings about a difficult subject.

Q & A

Question: What can I do about my mother? We are always fighting. She has so many rules and she snoops. I found her in my bedroom reading my diary.

Answer: It's not surprising that you are fighting more with your mom. Teens often feel a tension between their need for independence and their connection with their parents. For instance, you live in your parents' house and you're probably expected to abide by their rules, but you may not agree with all of those rules. In the same way, your mother may want you to become independent yet find it difficult to let go. It may be hard for her to accept that the child who once cried if she was lost in the supermarket is now dating, driving a car, and making decisions about life.

You can help your mother accept your independence by acting responsibly. Let her know that you are able to take care of yourself by doing it and doing it well. And don't be afraid to speak. Remind her that you still love her and you need her guidance every now and then, even if you don't need her to hold your hand when you cross the street anymore. Make some time for just you and her to do things that you've never had a chance to do before, like cooking dinner or going to see a movie. You may be surprised at what you discover about your mother—and yourself.

Arguments are an inevitable part of family life. Handled well, arguments can help family members learn about each other and grow closer. Learning to resolve differences with siblings can help them to develop the skills they'll need to have successful relationships with peers, teachers, coworkers, bosses, and spouses. Respectful, open discussions of conflicts can lead to greater intimacy between family members, even if family members cannot agree on the issues.

See also: Divorce and Families; Families, Divided; Teens in Trouble; Violence and the Family

FURTHER READING
Stone, Douglas, Bruce Patton, and Sheila Heen. *Difficult Conversations: How to Discuss What Matters Most.* New York: Penguin, 2000.
Weeks, Holly. *Failure to Communicate: How Conversations Go Wrong and What You Can Do to Right Them.* Boston: Harvard Business School Press, 2008.

■ BIRTH ORDER AND PSYCHOLOGY
The sequence in which siblings are born, where a person falls in that sequence, and the ways in which the order of one's birth affects emotional growth. Are you the "baby," the middle child, the older brother or sister? Or, perhaps you are somewhere in between in a larger family.

Birth order can be an important thing: Many experts agree that the order of birth is significant, because it can provide at least a hint about how brothers and sisters will develop psychologically as well as indicate what strengths and weaknesses they might have as they grow up. Sequence might even be instrumental in predicting who is more likely to succeed and who is more likely to struggle, and why.

People are like cards in a shuffled deck—we cannot choose when we appear nor how many cards are dealt before or after us. No matter how similar the cards may look on one side, they are very different on the flip side. Here is the trick: Many researchers believe that, if birth order is similar to dealing a deck of cards, science can begin to predict, based on when it is dealt, what card will appear. Perhaps we cannot predict the specific card, but at least we can expect a heart, a diamond, a club, or a spade.

This is not a universally accepted idea. Much other research challenges the idea, suggesting that birth order has little or no effect on a person's psychological development. Then there are only children (who tend to develop in a way similar to firstborn children); twins (because they are born simultaneously, the dynamic can be different for twins); and siblings in larger families (where roles can be much more complicated).

IS THERE A PATTERN?

Throughout history, cultures have assigned roles to children based on birth order, and there are numerous examples suggesting that firstborn children have an advantage over the brothers and sisters who follow them. However, it can be unfair to draw conclusions from such generalizations. In the language of statistics, it is important to know whether these examples are evidence of something real or just coincidences.

Time magazine explored the question in an article in October 2007. The writer noted that researchers from Norway, just a few months earlier, had released a study showing that firstborn children generally score higher on intelligence tests—as much as three points higher on an IQ test, compared to the scores of the next-oldest child. At the same time, the second child was about a point above the third child, the study showed. "While three points might not seem like much," the *Time* article noted, "the effect can be enormous. Just 2.3 IQ points can correlate to a 15-point difference in SAT scores [used in determining many college admissions], which makes an even bigger difference when you're an Ivy League applicant." The *Time* writer quotes a psychologist as saying, "In many families, the firstborn is going to get into Harvard and the second-born isn't."

That suggestion is not a new one. As early as 1874, a British scientist named Francis Galton published a study of 180 successful men and found that 99 of them were the firstborn sons in their families.

Other studies reached similar conclusions: One study of 314 eminent figures from the 1900s found that nearly 46 percent of them were firstborn children.

Time also reported that a poll of corporate leaders showed that 43 percent of top company officials are firstborn men and women; 33 percent had both older and younger siblings; and only 23 percent are the last-born in the family.

However, some of those same studies noted that success is hardly limited to firstborn siblings. There was evidence to suggest that while eldest children show some success in business and professional positions, younger brothers and sisters are more likely to become leaders who challenge authority, such as revolutionary leaders. Many become prominent scientists. Also, some studies show that younger siblings are more creative than firstborn children. In short, birth order is only

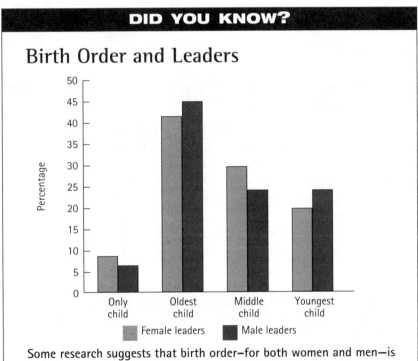

DID YOU KNOW?

Birth Order and Leaders

Some research suggests that birth order—for both women and men—is one way to predict success. However, it is far from foolproof, as many other studies show only minor variation.

Source: *Advancing Women* magazine (Winter 2001), at http://www.advancingwomen.com/awl/winter2001/zanville/Figures/figure4.gif.

one factor in determining whether a person has the potential to be a success.

HOW BIRTH ORDER AFFECTS US

In many cultures, the firstborn child–particularly (if unfairly) the firstborn son–is given a place of honor in the family. Even so, it is not all bad if you are not firstborn. Researchers suggest that boys and girls who are born later develop psychological tools to adapt and, often, to thrive better than their older siblings. Many develop a better sense of humor as a way of dealing with their status and as a way of winning favor from their parents and other adults. Others watch their older siblings and parents very closely and develop better strategies for dealing with stress, and ultimately for attaining success. Middle-born siblings, possibly owing to their position in the birth order, often develop excellent negotiating and peacemaking skills.

Q & A

Question: Why do firstborn sons seem to have an edge in finding success in school and careers?

Answer: There are many reasons, but back in the 1870s, the British scientist Francis Galton listed three good reasons. Firstborn sons, through the years, he said, are more likely to have the financial resources to continue their education. They also have the advantage of being "treated more as companions by parents," because they take some responsibility in helping raise their younger siblings. Finally, in low-income families, where food is in scarce supply, firstborn children usually get more attention and better nourishment.

Much of the discussion of birth order and its effect on psychological development can be traced back to the great early 20th-century psychiatrist Alfred Adler. He developed a broad overview of birth order and the personality and psychological traits that accompany the various positions in the family. He saw the only child as someone who likes to be the center of attention, especially among adults, and often struggles dealing with peers. The eldest child is authoritarian, enjoys power, but can be helpful to others. Sometimes a second child is more competitive, seeing the older sibling as a rival; sometimes a middle child is even-tempered but can struggle to find his or her place. The youngest child often has a special place in the family too and can develop big plans as a result.

It is easy to see what Adler was talking about—many people see themselves in his broad descriptions. Ultimately, though, just how important a role birth order plays in predicting personality warrants more study.

Dr. Robert Needlman, a pediatrician and author, has reviewed various studies and reached one conclusion that makes good sense: "Personality development," he wrote, "can't be distilled into a simple cookbook formula with birth order as the sole ingredient. But thinking about birth order can give you insight into how the forces within families shape children and the adults they grow up to become."

See also: Arguments and the Family; Family, The Traditional.

FURTHER READING
Leman, Kevin. *The Birth Order Book: Why You Are the Way You Are.* Grand Rapids, Mich.: Revell Books, 2004.

■ COMMUNICATION STYLES AND FAMILIES

The ways in which family members interact. Researchers have taken a close look at the way parents and children communicate, and they offer a great deal of help in figuring out what communication styles families use and which techniques can improve communication. Experts agree that family members need to think not only about what they say but also about the way they say it.

Perhaps the best way to think about communication styles is to think about everything that goes into delivering a message to someone in your family. Consider what you say when your mother asks what kind of day you had at school. You might say, "Just great." But were you smiling? Was it really a good day? Perhaps you rolled your eyes—that drastically changes the meaning of the words. Or maybe you let your mom catch a glance at your facial expression, hoping she will ask you more and invite you to tell her about a problem at school. In the two scenarios, the words you use—"Just great"—are exactly the same, but the message is very different.

In the same way, families can struggle to talk about things, both important and simple, just because they are having trouble sorting out all the hidden messages they believe they hear or see. It can be very frustrating. However, families can learn to communicate better simply by paying closer attention to just how they interact.

TEENS SPEAK

"I Finally Asked Her Why"

Our school day ends about 2:45, and I usually have something to do afterward. I'm in a few clubs, and I also play volleyball in the fall and soccer in the spring. Still, my mom says I have to be home for dinner at 5 P.M. sharp, no excuses. The same goes for all three of my brothers and sisters.

Sometimes, if we're home early, Mom will have us help cook, but she doesn't mind if we turn up exactly at five o'clock, just in time to sit down and eat. But if we're even five minutes late, she gets angry, and it usually means extra chores or even being grounded for a night. She really means it.

I never really understood why. One day, when I got into a conversation with friends and got home about 15 minutes late for dinner, Mom was angry and upset. I couldn't figure out why, so I asked her. She said, "It's the one time of the day when I can really find out what you and your brother and sisters are doing, and what you're thinking about. You're all so busy, and so am I." (She's a single mom and works two jobs.)

It's true—we rarely see each other since she leaves for her second job around 7:30 at night, when my aunt arrives to watch us. And rarely are all of us in the house together at the same time. Except at dinner.

I really like having dinner at home every day. And I'll be there on time tonight.

STYLES OF COMMUNICATION

In 1993, a group of researchers attempted to get to the heart of the matter by identifying four styles of communication that families use at different times, under different circumstances.

Clear and direct communication

The first style is clear and direct communication, which researchers consider to be the healthiest form of communication. In this style, a family member uses simple and plain language to deliver an honest message, such as a father's telling a son, "I am angry because I asked you to be home for dinner at five o'clock, and you came home an hour late; as a result, we all had to wait for you before we started to eat."

Clear and indirect communication

The second style is clear but indirect communication, which occurs when a clear message is delivered but not to the person for whom it is intended. For instance, in the example, the dad might turn to the mom at dinner and say, "This meatloaf is cold—it's too bad we couldn't eat at five o'clock like we planned, when it was hot." He might not have been talking to his son, but the son gets the message loud and clear.

Fact Or Fiction?

The most common way of communicating is talking to someone.

The Facts: Dr. William Petkanas, chair of the communications department at Western Connecticut State University, points out: "Much of our most important communication occurs in non-verbal languages, including gestures, tone, [and] facial expressions." Therefore, many of those "rules" are unspoken and unwritten, he notes, but everyone understands what they are, and, when they are violated, a person feels angry and betrayed. In short, the words alone are not the entire message: it is also how they are said.

Masked and direct communication

Researchers call the third category masked and direct communication, when the message is directed to the right person, but the message is less than clear. At dinner, for example, your dad might say to you upon your late arrival, "My father used to ground me when I disobeyed him." He is talking to you, but you might not be sure what he means by that remark, because he has not been clear. He has somewhat hidden, or masked, his meaning.

Masked and indirect communication

Finally, there is masked and indirect communication, in which both the message and its intended recipient are not clear. Perhaps your dad simply sighs, puts down his fork, and says to your mom, "The youth of today are just not reliable." This, researchers say, is the most unhealthy of the four types of communication.

When families communicate in this way, resentments build, confusion is common, misunderstandings are frequent, and small problems can turn into big ones—all because the family has simply failed to communicate effectively.

That is one way to describe the way families talk to each other, but there are certainly other ways to break it down, especially when it comes to negative tendencies. Some try to control the conversation and will not allow anyone else to talk, or will not listen in turn. Some refuse to talk at all, using the "silent treatment" to punish another family member. Some become emotional and will not allow a calm and clear discussion of real issues. All are learned behavior, and a family can often "unlearn" the damaging behavior and instead create an atmosphere where every family member feels comfortable speaking his or her mind, a place where everyone believes he or she is being heard.

Q & A

Question: What can families do to improve the way they communicate with each other?

Answer: Dr. Eric Maisel, a licensed marriage and family therapist and an author, says families need to learn to master "loving listening." *In 20 Communication Tips for Families,* he suggests these techniques:

1. Pay undivided attention when someone is speaking to you.

2. Be more interested in what is being said than in figuring out how to reply or fix the problem.

3. Wonder to yourself what is really going on. Use your powers of intuition and your lifetime of experience to understand what your parents or siblings are getting at. Plus, you can ask questions!

4. Take the time to listen, to consider what is being said, to gain clarity, and to frame direct but loving

responses. Communication takes time—and deserves the time it takes.

WHAT FAMILIES CAN DO

Families who want to improve how they interact with each other can do a few things to learn how to communicate better.

First, it is just a matter of communicating—a lot. Sometimes the most damaging thoughts are the ones left unsaid. However, it may seem harder to find the time to communicate effectively.

In an article for the Virginia Tech University Cooperative Extension, Professor Rick Peterson and graduate student Stephen Green note that a recent survey reported in the *Wall Street Journal* found that 40 percent of the people who responded said "lack of time was a greater problem for them than lack of money." They recommend that families set aside time to have meaningful conversation, whether it be around the breakfast or dinner table, in the car on the way to school, at bedtime, or at family meetings. The key is to make the time to talk and to use it.

Considering the four communication styles listed above, it is also important for families to make an effort to really say what they think—and to say it to the person who matters. Indirect communication just makes people frustrated and can lead to even bigger problems. Also, it is important to listen carefully to what people are saying and to try to be understanding. Watch for nonverbal clues indicating there might be more to the message than simply the words being spoken. Make sure you send positive cues back in return, by showing you really care about what is being said. Be sure to ask questions if you are confused about something.

Honesty and trust are important, and they must be in place for healthy communication to take place. At the same time, better communication usually will improve the level of honesty and trust in a family. More effective conversation is essential for a happy home life, and sometimes a little attention paid to how we say things, not just what we say, can go a long way toward keeping the peace.

See also: Arguments and the Family; Families, Blended; Families, Divided; Family Rules; Teens in Trouble; Violence and the Family.

FURTHER READING
Maisel, Eric. *20 Communication Tips for Families: A 30-Minute Guide to a Better Family Relationship.* Novato, Calif.: Pine Forge Press, 2000.

McKay, Gary D., and Steven A. Maybell. *Calming the Family Storm: Anger Management for Moms, Dads, and All the Kids.* Atascadero, Calif.: Impact Publishers, 2004.

■ DAY CARE

Day care is the provision of physical and emotional care to children while their parents or other caregivers are at work. Although the primary goal of day care is to provide for the needs of infants and young children, some providers may offer preschool education or after-school care for school-age children.

TYPES OF DAY CARE

Day care arrangements are classified by type. The three main types of day care described by the U.S. Census Bureau are care provided by relatives, family day care, and center-based care.

Day care provided by relatives involves an arrangement in which a family member other than a mother or father regularly cares for children. Parents either take the child to the relative's home, or the relative comes to the child's home for the hours the parents are away.

In family day care, the care is provided in the family residence of a provider. In some states, such a provider must attend an orientation and/or complete training to obtain a license. Regulatory requirements differ state to state. A provider might be approved, certified, registered, or licensed under state or local laws. California, for example, allows a provider to care for no more than four infants or six children without the help of an assistant. This regulation includes the provider's own children under the age of 12. With an assistant, the provider may care for 12 children; but no more than four may be infants, including their own children under the age of 12.

A third type of day care is center-based care, which involves the provision of care in a facility that is not part of a home. Centers may be in schools, churches, or company buildings and must meet specific health, safety, and other regulatory standards as outlined by specific states. The staff of day care centers are trained and credentialed in early childhood development and education.

ALTERNATIVES TO DAY CARE

The U.S. Census Bureau reports smaller numbers of parents choosing alternatives to the three main types of day care. One alternative is to form a neighborhood day care cooperative. According to Jane Filstrup in the book *Monday through Friday: Day Care Alternatives,* every parent in the cooperative provides care to a group of children for an agreed-upon number of days per month.

Another alternative is to hire a live-in nanny, governess, or au pair to tend to the children. An au pair is a young man or woman, often from another country, who lives with a family while caring for their children. This day care alternative is costly and not usually an option for mid- to low-income families.

AN EXPENSIVE SERVICE

According to *Parents and the High Price of Child Care: 2009 Update,* published by the National Association of Child Care Resource and Referral Agencies (NACCRRA), studies indicate that in 2008, 63 percent of the nation's children under five years of age were in some type of weekly child care arrangement. The highest average cost for full-time day care was $11,680 annually. Part-time care was relatively more expensive, with the highest average cost reported to be $10,720 per year. Average prices differed among different age groups of children. Infant care was reported as high as $10,324, $9,805 for four-year-olds, and school-age children cost $7,124 annually. The cost for day care were higher than the cost of food each month. In families with two children, the monthly day care costs were more than the family spent on rent and about the same as they spent on the home mortgage payment.

IS IT WORTH THE COST?

In the 2009 update of *Parents and the High Price of Child Care,* findings also indicated that American families as of 2008 in 33 states and the District of Columbia spent annually more on their preschooler's day care than on the annual tuition at a four-year public university.

FINANCIAL ASSISTANCE

Provided by the State of America's Children 2008, the report *Early Childhood Care and Development* delivers on government financial assistance for day care. Results show 1 million families receive child care assistance. Eligibility for assistance is based on income ranges. In Missouri, for example, eligibility is just above the poverty line, whereas it is as high as 275 percent above the poverty line in Maine. If day care for children was provided for all families with an income less than 200 percent of the federal poverty line, it is estimated by the Urban Institute that 2.7 million people would be lifted out of poverty. In 2008, this was equivalent to $35,200 for a family of three.

NUMBER OF HOURS CHILDREN ARE IN DAY CARE PER WEEK

In 2008, *The NICHID Study of Early Child Care and Youth Development* showed that between the ages of three months and one and a half years, 27 percent of children were in day care for a minimum of 10 hours per week. Thirty-seven percent of these children were in day care for more than 30 hours per week. In children between the ages of one and a half and 3 years, 44 percent were in day care for more than 30 hours per week. Fifty percent of children three to four and a half were in child care for more than 30 hours each week.

ADVANTAGES FOR CHILDREN IN DAY CARE

The 2008 NICHID report also examined the relationship between the amount of day care a child is exposed to and his or her developmental outcomes. Children ages one and a half, two, three and four and a half were assessed. Results indicated that the amount of time a child spent in day care was not associated with his or her cognitive or language skills nor a child's ability to enter school. Also in 2008, the *B. E. Journal of Economic Analysis & Policy* published a study that used a nationally representative sample of children to examine the relationship between after-school supervision and cognitive achievement. The study measured the effects of family and nonfamily supervision to determine if a difference existed. The results showed that whether by a family member or nonfamily member, adult supervision was not related to a child's cognitive performance. However, family member supervision was related to improved cognitive performance as a result of personal or family-specific traits. It was not found that nonfamily member adult supervision led to lower cognitive outcomes however.

Socialization-related advantages of day care are that children learn to relate to those who are not the same age, advises the Office for Young Children, a child-care resource group. Interactions with older children and teachers provide modeling behavior for children along with opportunities for additional social skill development.

The Children's Defense Fund states that additional advantages of day care include improved nutrition, health screening, and access to early childhood related services for children and families.

Q & A

Question: Do day care centers provide care to children with special learning, medical, or behavioral needs?

Answer: According to the Americans with Disabilities Act, family day care and center-based day care centers must offer child care to children with disabilities. The only exception to this law relates to centers run directly by religious organizations. In the United States, the government does not legislate the policies and procedures of faith-based agencies.

SEPARATION ISSUES

The research related to attachment and separation issues in young children is contradictory. Positive outcomes related to cognitive development for children in day care are well documented by child advocacy agencies such as the Children's Defense Fund and by government agencies such as the National Institute of Child Health and Human Development. But noted experts T. Berry Brazelton and Stanley Greenspan raise concerns about young children in day care. In their well-respected book *The Irreducible Needs of Children,* they explore the critical needs of young children, especially infants, and question children's ability to bond well emotionally when in day care for long periods of time without consistent nurturing care providers.

Fact Or Fiction?

A child will be less upset if his mother leaves day care while he is busy playing than if she tells him she is leaving.

The Facts: Separation issues are a key concern related to the emotional well-being of young children. Brazelton and Greenspan's review of research on attachment suggests children separate more effectively when they are prepared for the separation and placed in the care of nurturing, well-trained care providers. When parents leave without warning, separation issues may be made worse. When separation is handled with honesty and compassion, children can learn to trust care providers and that parents will return.

However, the 2008 NICHID *Study of Early Child Care and Youth Development,* as well as a 2000 report "The Impact of Day Care on Child Development" by the psychologist Ercilia Palacio-Quintin, shows little negative effect, on development and well-being, even if children attend full time and are enrolled at young ages. The primary indicator of emotional well-being, researchers say, is having a secure attachment to a consistent caregiver.

Research evidence does not suggest that day care per se is detrimental to children's future social and emotional development. The separation and attachment concerns center on whether or not children receive nurturing and consistent care either at home or in day care.

DAY CARE ISSUES AND CONCERNS

Equal access to quality, affordable day care remains an issue for families, day care providers, and regulatory agencies. The issues and concerns surrounding day care are related to availability of day care, safety, health, and staffing.

Availability

In some areas, the biggest issue surrounding day care is that there isn't enough of it. For example, in some communities in California, there are not enough day care centers for all the children needing day care. According to the Marin Child Care Council, as many as 15 percent of all children of working parents in Marin county don't have access to care.

Safety

While safety standards may be clearly outlined by each state, compliance with these regulations continues to be an issue. The Florida Department of Children and Families, a group that inspects Florida centers to ensure child safety, found in their years of ongoing monitoring that some centers continue to use vans without car seats or seat belts. Some vans were uninsured and had no schedule for safety inspections. Monitoring activities also revealed centers that use drivers without licenses.

Safety standards are outlined federally by such organizations as the National Association for the Education of Young Children, the National Health and Safety Performance Standards, the American Academy of Pediatrics, and the American Public Health Association. The report, "State Efforts to Enforce Safety and Health Requirements," found that states often met or exceeded the federal standards. Yet the ability for states to inspect and support compliance with the regulations was found to be problematic.

Health problems
Children in day care get more illnesses than children who are cared for at home. Studies reviewed by Palacio-Quintin show that the illness rate is as much as two to four times higher for children in day care. Many of the illnesses are mild health concerns such as colds, flu, and stomach and intestinal problems. Yet, some illnesses are more concerning such as measles, whooping cough, pneumonia, and cytomegalovirus (CMV). Communicable diseases are spread when sick children are in close contact with one another and when staff members and children inadequately wash hands after coming in contact with urine, feces, saliva, or nasal secretions.

Staffing difficulties
The three critical staff difficulties in day care centers are turnover, **staff ratio,** and untrained workers. The Center for the Childcare Workforce, in 2002, explored salaries, benefits, and turnover rates in day care centers throughout the United States. The average yearly turnover rate was 21 percent; some centers had a turnover rate as high as 51 percent. The Bureau of Labor Statistics reported in 2008 that child day care services provided about 859,200 wage and salary jobs in 2008. Also in 2008, hourly earnings of nonsupervisory workers in the child day care services industry averaged $11.32, much less than the average of $18.08 throughout private industry. On a weekly basis, earnings in child day care services averaged only $345 in 2008, compared with the average of $608 in private industry. According to the Center for the Child Care Workforce, the mean hourly wage for child care workers in 2007 was $9.32, approximately $18,623 per year. As reported by the Early Child Care Research Center, salaries are a good measure of staff stability; when salaries are high, caregivers stay.

Staff ratio refers to the number of children per staff member. The National Institute of Child Health and Human Development recommends staff ratios of 1:4 for infants and 1:7 for preschoolers. In both family day care and center-based day care, sensitive, responsive, and individualized interactions with children are the best measures of quality care. There is a direct relationship between appropriate staff ratios and staff being able to provide quality care. But providing better ratios is expensive. Day care agencies that strive to achieve better ratios must hire more employees, and more employees means more money spent on salaries and benefits.

DAY CARE IN THE FUTURE

Increasing numbers of parents are joining the workforce, according to the U.S. Census Bureau, and a growing body of research points to the need for quality, affordable day care for children. Child-development experts, advocates, and policy makers put forward a call to action regarding day care in the annual report, *The State of America's Children,* which discusses ways in which day care can be improved in the future. The three areas where the most impact might be made are in funding, availability of day care, and in curriculum development.

Funding and availability

The goal of improving day care funding methods should be broad-based. Although there is now some subsidized care, the ideal would be more subsidized care, to cover all eligible children. Experts and advocates call on government leaders to invest in the funding of quality day care aimed at bridging the serious gap of its availability. The Children's Defense Fund recommends adequate funding to meet the goals of providing early learning skills for young children especially those from poor families as well as providing after-school programs.

Curriculum development

Research-based and developmentally appropriate curricula should be the goal of every day care provider. According to family studies professor Dianna Chiabotti of Napa Valley College, teachers with training and education in child development provide quality care to children. The standard to attain is that all centers be accredited, and to have workers receive ongoing training.

Developmentally appropriate curricula are those in which children are exposed to information, language and social experiences that encourage a love of learning.

See also: Financial Management, Marital; Single-Parent Families

FURTHER READING

Chaudry, Ajay. *Putting Children First: How Low-Wage Working Mothers Manage Childcare.* New York: Russell Sage Foundation Publications, 2006.

Galinsky, Ellen. *Mind in the Making: The Seven Essential Life Skills Every Child Needs.* New York: HarperCollins, 2010.

■ DEATH IN THE FAMILY

A death in the family means the loss of a family member and may include the loss of a child or an adult. According to statistics reported in 2006 by The Compassionate Friends (TCF), a national organization that aids grieving families, more than 150,000 infants, children, teens, and young adults die each year; 900,000 families experience the loss of a child in early pregnancy and in 2009, about 27,000 faced a still-birth (an infant delivered without signs of life).

Families face the death of a loved one in many ways because every family has a different social network and engages in different rituals. These differences mean that although a death in a family is a universal event, each family copes with the loss in its own way.

The death of a relative affects everyone in the family, both young and old. It may also cause stresses in the family, as the household changes in response to the loss. There is a similarity, however, in the way adults and children grieve.

BEREAVEMENT

Bereavement is sadness about the loss of a loved one. When a death occurs in a family, the sadness experienced by both the adults and children is often a complex feeling with many responses.

Adult response to grief

When adults lose a parent, a spouse, a sibling, or a child, they may be unable, at first, to accept that their loved one is gone. Some become so depressed that they are unable to make the necessary life adjustments. The Compassionate Friends finds that when adults lose a parent, they often feel as if they have lost a part of their past. When they lose a spouse, they often feel they have lost the present, and when they lose a child, they often feel they have lost the future. TCF finds that adults who lose a sibling feel as if potentially the longest relationship of their life has ended. In this way, a sibling's death can seem like the loss of the past, present, and the future.

Among the feelings individuals experience after a family member dies are sadness, anger, anxiety, depression, and fear of being alone.

Some people withdraw from friends, lose interest in eating, have trouble sleeping, or become irritable.

A landmark 1985 study in the journal *Social Work* underscored the particular strain that a child's death places on parents. Researcher T. Rando found that eventually 80 percent of these bereaved parents divorced.

Children's response to grief

Children respond to a death in the family in ways characteristic of their age. According to the Royal College of Psychiatrists in a guide titled "Death in the Family: Helping Children Cope," infants often become anxious because they pick up on the feelings of the adults around them. Infants know their routine has been altered; as a result, they may become hard to settle. Some preschoolers view death as temporary, even reversible. Young children may think that they caused the death and are therefore to blame. They may revert to behaviors more typical of younger children, experience nightmares, develop issues with toileting, or may talk about their loved one or imitate this person.

According to the guide, older children, by contrast, know that death is permanent. They know that someone who is deceased can no longer be heard or seen. They also know that all living beings die and death has a cause. Teens, the guide notes, may have intense feelings about a loss but may not show them openly. They may not be able to put their feelings into words or may be reluctant to upset others. Even though they may not show that they are upset, many teens grieve deeply. Each teen's response is unique, based on his or her personality. One teen may withdraw and feel lost, while another may feel angry. Older children may have issues with grades and friendships; some may refuse to go to school at all.

Some teens may be frightened by feelings of grief and may resist the grief process. The Dougy Center, which has provided support for more than 13,500 bereaved families, has found that teens deal with grief in constructive ways by writing about their feelings in a journal or confiding in trusted friends. Some teens try to escape the pain of a loss through substance abuse, careless sexual activity, skipping school, and engaging in other risky behaviors. These ways of handling grief have destructive outcomes.

Children of all ages may display feelings of loss sporadically over a long period of time. Parents may see anger or sadness related to the loss continue on and off for years.

Comforting children

Parents do best when they tell their children about a death and answer their questions simply and honestly. After a review of the research, the Neuropsychiatric Institute at the University of California concluded that even very young children understand that something terrible has happened when a parent dies or is seriously ill even if they are not told directly. By withholding this information, adults fail to protect children and provide age-appropriate support.

According to Dr. Alan Greene of the Stanford University School of Medicine, children as early as three who experience a loss can be encouraged to express their feelings through play or by drawing pictures, using puppets, or making up a story. Elementary school children may dramatize their feelings as a way of working through grief.

The Dougy Center advises parents to tell children when and where the funeral will be, who will attend, and what will happen at the ceremony. Children should be asked if they wish to attend. Some children view the funeral as a chance to say goodbye to the deceased. If they do not want to go to the funeral, however, they should not be forced to attend. There are other ways that children can be involved, says Greene. For example, parents can take the children later to visit the gravesite. They might light a candle together, say a prayer, or tell each other what the person meant in their lives.

Adults who wish to comfort a teen need to first sort out their own feelings so that they can better relate as companions in grief. The Center advises against lecturing a teen about the proper way to grieve. Instead it recommends listening and then offering constructive ideas about facing sadness. Teens will want to work through the process of grieving in their own unique ways, which should be honored by adults.

Fact Or Fiction?

When a family loses a loved one in tragic circumstances such as in an accident or through suicide, the family will never be the same again.

The Facts: Families can grieve in healthy ways and go on to live productive, happy lives, no matter the circumstances of the loss. When families communicate with each other clearly and often about the loss, healthy grieving occurs. It is important for each person to accept the death and for family members to share with each other an acceptance of the new reality of family life. Families who grieve in healthy ways recognize that the death is permanent and means permanent changes to family structure and function. While the loss is never forgotten, healthy grief work includes a reorganization of family. Members begin to seek out new relationships and life pursuits.

ROLE OF RELIGION IN GRIEVING

Religious beliefs and participation in worship services play a role in the way families grieve. Ceremonies, customs, and rituals allow families to grieve with the support of other relatives and friends, and give grieving relatives time to remember or pray for the deceased.

When death occurs in a family, relatives and friends need to grieve. Everyone associated with the loss is touched in his or her own way. Coming together at religious ceremonies helps those who are grieving to celebrate the life of the loved one as well as find meaning in life and loss. At different ages, people react differently to the death of a loved one. Although grief stresses the family, there are ways that families can cope and can comfort children. Religious customs aim to assist families through the process of coming to terms with loss.

Q & A

Question: Why do families put themselves through a wake and funeral? These rituals seem only to make people more upset.

Answer: The rituals of wakes and funerals allow people the opportunity to express deep feelings among others who care for and about them and the person who died. Often these religious rituals and ceremonies also provide family and friends a chance to express their feelings and receive support from members of a person's faith community.

See also: Family Traditions; Religion and the Family

FURTHER READING

Myers, Edward. *Teens, Loss, and Grief: The Ultimate Teen Guide.* It Happened to Me. No. 8. Lanham, Md.: Scarecrow Press, 2006.

Walukonis, Jodi A. *Griping About Grief, A Teen's Navigation Through the Loss of a Loved One.* Sarasota, Fla.: Peppertree Press, 2007.

Wolfelt, Alan D. *Twelve Critical Questions for Mourners . . .: The Answers That Will Help You Heal.* Fort Collins, Colo.: Center for Loss & Life Transition, 2010.

■ DIVORCE AND FAMILIES

Divorce is the legal ending of a marriage. During the process of a divorce, a couple's property and debts are divided. If children are involved, their **custody** and care are decided. In some cases, a former spouse may be required to provide financial support to the other, either permanently or temporarily. After the divorce is finalized, each individual can legally marry someone else.

SEPARATION ISSUES

The first step toward divorce is **separation.** Separation means moving out, starting a different household, and changing routine. Most states require that people live in separate households for a designated period of time before divorcing. When couples decide to separate, parents and children may experience emotional turmoil including depression, loneliness, and other feelings of grief. Coping is hardest when one partner wants to divorce and the other does not, if the idea is sudden and unexpected, or when friends and family members disapprove.

In addition to the emotional pain of separation, families must make many practical decisions. Who will stay and who will leave? Where will family members live? How will assets and debts be divided? Who will pay for what, now and in the future? If the couple has children, will the children live with one parent or the other? How will they share time between parents? Who will pay the children's expenses?

Marital therapists sometimes recommend that couples try a structured separation for a limited period of time before making a final decision about a divorce. During a structured separation, the couple stops living together. Partners attend regularly scheduled therapy sessions with a professional therapist and see each other at specified times. Because it puts couples in a new environment, separation may interrupt old patterns of interaction.

Trial separations may be useful for couples who are not sure if they want to divorce or in cases where there is extreme conflict between partners, including physical and verbal abuse. A separation may allow a cooling-off period of personal growth and freedom while the couple works to restructure the relationship. Stressful life events, such as the loss of a job, death of a loved one, change in jobs, relocation, or children leaving home often bring out problems in a marriage. Separation may allow the partner experiencing the stress to deal with the crisis apart from the problems in the marriage. When partners are simply unable to decide whether to divorce or not, a structured separation may help them to make a decision.

Most separations end with divorce or the couple reuniting. However, some couples choose to remain married but legally separated, either for religious or other reasons. In these cases, the legal obligations of the marriage end but no divorce occurs. Couples who are separated but not divorced must negotiate issues including child custody, finances, and maintaining separate households, but they cannot remarry unless they eventually decide to divorce.

SPLIT FAMILIES

For children of divorced parents, divorce often means living with a semi-packed suitcase, spending weekends with one parent and weekdays with the other. It may mean new friends, moving to a new home, attending a new school, and dealing with parents who are angry with one another. Economic hardship is common after a divorce, especially for families headed by women. In a 2002 study of the economic impact of family structure on children, economists Marianne E. Page and Ann Huff Stevens found that divorced parents experienced a 41 percent decline in family income in the year following a divorce. Family food consumption falls by 18 percent in the year following divorce. Using a dynamic model with longitudinal effects, Page and Huff calculated that six years later, children whose parents remained unmarried had family incomes of 45 percent lower than if the divorce had not occurred.

Divorcing families often must decide who will have **custody** or **guardianship** of the children. There are two types of custody: **physical custody** and **legal custody.** Physical custody defines where the child will live. The child might split his or her time between parents, or he or she may live with one parent and visit the other. Legal custody determines who will make decisions about how the child is raised. These decisions include medical care, religious upbringing, and schooling. These types of custody may be given to one or to both parents. If one parent has **sole custody,** he or she has both physical and legal custody of the child. Usually, the other parent has visitation rights. In **joint custody,** parents share physical and legal custody.

If parents cannot agree about custody of the children, they may seek help from a **mediator.** A mediator is a person who usually has a background in law or the behavioral sciences and specializes in helping couples resolve the issues that arise in a divorce. In other cases, a judge may appoint a child development expert to investigate the family situation and make recommendations about custody.

Decisions about custody are made on the basis of what is best for the child, instead of assuming that the child will stay with the mother. Still, most children of divorced parents live with their mothers. In 2007, according to the U.S. Census Bureau, 83 percent of the 13.6 million custodial parents were women.

When a family splits, older children may find themselves taking on more responsibility. Without two adults to share the tasks of keeping the home and earning a living, some responsibilities may fall on children. Teens especially may find themselves helping with cooking, cleaning the house, and even earning extra money to help support the family. Children may find it difficult to adjust to the constraints of a lower income and not being able to buy things that they were once able to afford.

Fact Or Fiction?

Parents feel differently toward their children after a divorce.

The Facts: Immediately after a divorce, parents may be more involved in their own concerns and needs and be less attentive to their children. They may still be dealing with their own grief and pain at the dissolution of the relationship with their spouse. After divorce, parents may spend less time with their children, simply because each parent must work more hours to maintain a household. But this does not mean their feelings for their children have changed. It may seem that parents feel differently toward their children after a divorce, but this is rarely, if ever, true.

DIFFICULT DIVORCE AND KIDS

Only rarely is a divorce not marked by conflict. Often, tension and arguments between parents continue even after the former spouses have gone their separate ways. When parents cannot manage their anger at each other and bring their children into the struggle, children are torn between the two most important people in their lives.

Researchers continue to debate about the long-term effects of divorce and parental conflict on children. Some, such as psychologist Judith Wallerstein, argue that parental divorce has long-term negative effects on children's growth and development. In a 30-year study, from 1971 to 2001, of 60 divorced families in Marin County, California, involving 130 children, Wallerstein found that 10 years after divorce, 50 percent of the women and 33 percent of the men were still angry at their ex-partners and that this anger affected their relationships with their children. Memories of abandonment, terror, and loneliness were common among the children in Wallerstein's study. Many felt that they had been denied basic security while growing up and that they had "lost" their childhood by feeling the need to take care of their parents.

The negative effects seemed to grow worse over time. Ten to 15 years later, many of the children in the study had a record of illegal offenses, had engaged in sexual activity with multiple partners, and had abused alcoholic beverages. As they entered adulthood, half the children were underachieving. Financial support was limited and few had the resources to go to college. Wallerstein concluded that divorce causes serious harm to children who experience it.

Wallerstein's study, however, did not look at how children are affected by the conflict prior to divorce. The results of several other studies suggest that marital conflict has a greater effect on children's well-being than the divorce itself. For example, in 1991, sociologists Paul Amato and Alan Booth of the Population Research Center at Pennsylvania State University published "Parental Divorce and the Wellbeing of Children: A Meta-Analysis." Amato and Booth combined the results of 129 studies involving 95,000 participants. They compared children whose parents divorced to those whose parents remained married. They found that there were often problems in parent-child relationships eight to 12 years before the divorce. The lower the quality of the parents' marriage, the less close the parents were to their children at the age 18. Fathers and children were less affectionate toward each other after divorce, suggesting that the relationship between parents and children was impacted both directly and indirectly.

In 2001, Joan B. Kelly, a psychiatrist at the University of California at San Francisco, published "Adjustment in Conflicted Marriage and Divorce," a review of research on the impact of marital conflict, parental violence, and divorce on the psychological adjustment of children.

Kelly looked at studies that had been published during the 1990s. She also found that parental conflict, not the separation of parents, has the strongest negative impact on children's well-being. Her summary of the research on children and divorce supports the idea that children's emotional or behavioral problems may arise from conflict between parents, before and after the divorce, more than from the divorce itself.

Kelly also notes that teens who are caught in the middle of their parents' post-divorce disagreements tend to have more problems adjusting than those whose parents do not use their children to express their conflicts. Kelly explains that, for teens, being "caught in the middle" might mean being asked to relay angry messages or requests or spy on a parent. Such children often feel the need to hide their feelings and thoughts about the other parent.

In 2009, researchers published findings in the journal *Child Abuse & Neglect*. The data used for the study was taken from a national sample of 5,877 individuals ranging in age from 15 to 54 years. The study examined the affect of parental divorce on the development of psychiatric problems in children. The results showed that parental divorce was associated with mental health problems. Another 2009 study explored the association between parental divorce and adolescent drunkenness. The sample included 3,694 elementary school students. The results showed parental divorce had a strong influence on increasing the likelihood of drunkenness in children.

Some high-conflict post-divorce families can benefit from working with a **parenting coordinator.** A parenting coordinator works within the structure of a couple's divorce decree to help parents settle disagreements about children, and can facilitate between parents who are in high conflict. Visits should always be supervised if conflict threatens a child's well-being, if there is a risk of physical threat and abuse between parents, or if physical or sexual abuse of children is a possibility.

TEENS SPEAK

Surviving My Parents' Divorce

I had just returned home from soccer practice on a Sunday afternoon late in August when Dad called my younger brother Jeremy and me down to the kitchen. He looked so serious. My first thought was, "We must be in big trouble." Mom was sitting at the table. I could tell that she had been crying. Her mascara was in streaks down her face. That's when Dad told us that he was moving to an apartment about four miles away, and he and Mom were getting divorced. He would be leaving the next day.

It wasn't entirely a surprise. Mom and Dad had been fighting for a long time. I still have a picture of all of us, taken when my little brother was about a year old. I was four. We were at the beach near our house. Mom, Jeremy, and I were burying Dad in the sand, and he was laughing. We all looked so happy in the picture. For at least three years, I had wondered what happened to that smiling, laughing Mom and Dad in the picture. I know they tried not to fight in front of us, but still, we heard the angry voices.

The next few months were horrible. Dad moved out and Mom cried a lot. We visited Dad on weekends. It felt strange to go to his apartment and sleep on the couch in the living room. Mom started shopping at thrift stores for my clothes. I was so embarrassed. I was sure that everyone at school could tell that my clothes had come from the Salvation Army store. I was angry at her for not buying me things at department stores. Then one day, when we were at the grocery store, she didn't have enough money to pay for all the groceries. That was when I realized that she was not just being mean— she was barely able to pay for our food and other things we needed. She was going to college, and Dad had lost his job, so she wasn't receiving child support payments.

After about a year, Dad got a new job and moved to Oregon. Mom finished school, and she is an accountant at a busy office. Jeremy and I spend summers with Dad and the rest of the year with Mom in California. I still wish they hadn't split up, but I know that it was the best thing for all of us. I've gotten closer to each of them, and I've learned that I can survive really tough times.

AMICABLE DIVORCE AND KIDS

While post-divorce conflict is common, hostility between parents usually lessens dramatically after divorce. In a 1999 study of the effects of nonresident father visitation and conflict on children, Valarie King and Holly E. Heard found that three years after divorcing, only 8–12 percent of divorced couples remained in very high conflict. King and Heard analyzed data from 1,565 mothers living with children under the age of 18 years whose fathers lived elsewhere.

For children of divorce, the relatively quick lessening of hostility between parents is good news. As Kelly notes, many studies show that children whose divorced parents cooperate and mutually support each other are more likely to adjust well emotionally, psychologically, and socially. A 2009 study determined parental hostility or conflict has more negative influence on children than parental divorce. According to this study, sibling relationship quality is lower in families that experience a higher level of hostility between parents. Parental divorce was shown to improve relationships among siblings in these families. In low-conflict families, the impact of parental divorce on sibling relationships was not significant. Many divorcing families have found that professional assistance such as postmarital therapy or divorce mediation helps them resolve disputes amicably, even in the early stages of divorce.

A mediator helps the couple develop a written agreement that serves as the basis of the divorce petition to the court, according to Kelly. The divorce petition spells out how the couple will divide their assets, child custody, and visitation rights; who will pay child support and how much it will be; and other workings of the divorce. Mediation emphasizes open communication, negotiation, and mutual resolution of the emotional, financial, and child-related issues. Of couples who used mediation, at least 40 percent were able to completely agree on the terms of their divorce and up to 80 percent were able to agree on at least some points. Many couples who participated in mediation say that it helped them focus on the needs of their children, gave them a chance to express their feelings and grievances, and allowed them to deal with fundamental issues in greater depth than would occur in court procedures.

Kelly notes that many studies indicate that children do better when they have a close relationship with their noncustodial parent (usually the father). According to Kelly, the frequency and pattern of contacts between fathers are related to marital and post-divorce conflict and the amount of legal conflict. She cites the work of Paul Amato and colleagues, who found that children adjusted most easily when they had frequent contact with their nonresident fathers and conflict between their divorced parents was low.

King and Heard found that the mother's satisfaction with the father's visits was a key indicator of the child's well-being. In their study, the more satisfied mothers were with the fathers' visit, the more satisfied they were overall. When mothers were dissatisfied, children had more behavioral problems and scored lower than other children on tests of adjustment and well-being. This was true even if fathers visited frequently.

In "Children of Divorce," a review of recent medical literature about children of divorce, Charles Bryner, a naval physician, observes that both children and adults experience divorce in a series of stages. These stages, argues Bryner, are similar to those Elisabeth Kübler-Ross described for terminally ill patients: denial, anger, bargaining, depression, and acceptance. However, these stages may be experienced differently by children and adults. When adults are too preoccupied with their own sorrow at the ending of the relationship, children may be forgotten and remain stuck in the denial stage.

Bryner offers the following summary of children's common feelings and actions during these five stages. During the denial stage, children often believe that their parents will reunite, a fantasy that can persist for years. In the second stage, anger, children may feel furious at their parents for not trying harder to stay together and allowing the divorce to happen. They may feel that their parents have ruined their lives and destroyed their vision of the future. In the bargaining stage, children may try to bring the absent parent home by being "perfect." They may try to get good grades at school, go out of their way to be helpful, and not cause any trouble. Young children may believe that their own misbehaviors caused their parents' divorce (for example, fighting with a sibling). A period of extreme sadness and tiredness, or **depression,** usually follows the bargaining period. The child often feels sad, tired, and listless both at school and at home. For children to move on to the final stage, acceptance, they must develop the emotional maturity and distance to recognize that their parents are happier living separately and that the divorce was in the best interests of all family members. Acceptance often does not occur until adolescence or even young adulthood.

While divorce is a stressful and painful occurrence for families, most children do eventually adjust to their parents' divorce and go on to lead happy, fulfilling lives. In *For Better or for Worse: Divorce Reconsidered,* psychologist E. Mavis Hetherington and colleague John Kelly report the results of a 24-year study of 1,400 families begun in the late 1970s. Six years after their parents' divorce, almost 80 percent of the children whose parents had divorced were as happy and as emotionally healthy as those whose parents were still together.

DIVIDING UP DAYS: WHEN DO WE SEE WHOM?

One of the most difficult decisions for most divorcing families is where children will live and whether one or both parents will care for them. Even when parents share joint legal and physical custody, it may not be practical, or best for their child, to evenly split their time between homes (for example, spending three days a week at the mother's house and four days at the father's). Geography, work schedules, and other factors all play a role in determining when and how children spend time with which parent. Each family must create custody arrangements appropriate for both parents and children. Some experts prefer the term *co-parenting* as a more accurate description of shared parental responsibilities. Arrangements, such as spending school years with Dad and summers with Mom, might be more practical for a particular family. The child's age, social network, and other needs should be taken into account when deciding who spends time with whom. Older children and teens should be active participants in choosing how and where they want to spend their time.

Holidays, birthdays, and other days of traditional celebration can create chaos in split families. Parents who share the same religion may both want to share the same holidays with their children. Children's birthdays and school vacations may be another source of conflict. Like any other aspect of post-marital family life, disputes over holidays and special occasions can be worked out amicably or can become another source of conflict. Many parents have developed workable solutions that allow everyone to share in the celebrations of these special days (for example, alternating Christmas Eve and Christmas Day). Birthdays may be celebrated twice, once with each parent. School and work vacations can be divided up in ways that work for everyone. Children, especially teens and older children, should participate in these decisions.

See also: Arguments and the Family; Families, Blended; Families, Divided; Family, The New; Family, The Traditional; Marriage and Family, Changes in; Single-Parent Families; Stepparents; Violence and the Family

FURTHER READING

Brotherton, M. *Split: A Graphic Reality Check for Teens Dealing with Divorce.* Sisters, Oreg.: Multhomah Publishers, 2006.

Jones, Jami L. *Bouncing Back: Dealing With the Stuff Life Throws at You.* London: Franklin Watts, 2007.

Schab, Lisa M. *The Divorce Workbook for Teens: Activities to Help You Move Beyond the Breakup.* Oakland, Calif.: New Harbinger Publications Inc., 2008.

Trueit, Trudi S. *Surviving Divorce: Teens Talk About What Hurts and What Helps.* London: Franklin Watts, 2007.

■ ELDERLY FAMILY MEMBERS

Parents or grandparents during late adulthood are considered to be elderly. Adults age 65–74 are sometimes referred to as the young-old, those age 75–84 as the middle-old, and those 85 and older as the oldest-old.

Late adulthood is often a time of transition from independence to **physical dependence** on others for activities such as walking, bathing, taking medications, or balancing a checkbook. The scale used to measure a person's ability to perform physical tasks is called the **Activities of Daily Living** (ADL). During late adulthood, physical health may deteriorate to the point where seniors are no longer able to care for themselves. According to the 2007 American Community Survey (ACS), conducted by the U.S. Census Bureau, almost half (43 percent) of people age 65 or older had at least one disability, physical or nonphysical. Among people age 75 or older, more than one-half (55 percent) were living with at least one disability.

While many disabilities are minor, others may interfere with one's independence. The need for assistance with ADLs increases drastically with age. Data from the 2007 survey show that 4.7 percent of people age 65–74 experienced difficulty caring for themselves, as did 6.8 percent of those age 75–84 and 11.7 percent of those older than 85. As people move from the middle-old to the oldest-old group, the need for highly personalized care, such as assistance using the toilet or bathing, becomes three times more common.

NURSING HOMES

Many elderly people who have great difficulty performing ADLs enter nursing homes, special residential facilities that offer skilled nursing

DID YOU KNOW?

Life Expectancy in the United States by Ethnicity and Gender

Measure and Sex	Both Races 2006	Both Races 2005	White 2006	White 2005	Black 2006	Black 2005
Life expectancy at birth	77.1	77.4	78.2	77.9	73.2	72.8
Male	75.1	74.9	75.7	75.4	69.7	69.3
Female	80.2	79.9	80.6	80.4	76.5	76.1

Source: National Center for Health Statistics, 2009.

care. They are designed to care for people who need high levels of assistance with medical and personal care such as the administration of medications, moving around, or personal hygiene. Data from the 2008 American Community Survey showed that almost 1.6 million people in the United States—4.5 percent of the population age 65 and over—lived in nursing homes.

Fact Or Fiction?

All elderly people have serious disabilities that cause them to require daily assistance.

The Facts: Many of the elderly lead active, independent lives. Some continue to work, either full- or part-time, past the age of 65. Others use their retirement years to travel, pursue volunteer activities, hobbies, and other interests.

Nursing homes vary greatly in cost and quality. Many are clean, well-run facilities that offer caring, compassionate assistance to residents. These high-quality nursing homes have well-trained, professional staff that includes nurses, physicians, dietitians, physical therapists, and other licensed or certified health care providers. These facilities have safety features such as wheelchair ramps, nonskid floor coverings, grab bars in hallways and bathrooms, fire alarms, and sprinkler systems. Some residents are moderately active, even if the activity is sitting in a chair. Other residents must remain in bed all day, but they are dressed and well groomed. Well-run nursing homes also offer recreational activities, as well as healthy, attractive foods at meals. Residents have privacy for phone calls, visits of family and friends, and personal care such as bathing or dressing. They are allowed to decorate their rooms with their personal belongings. However, these facilities can be extremely costly, and private or public health insurance programs such as Medicaid or Medicare may not cover those costs.

When considering whether to place an elderly parent in a nursing home, adult children should inspect any prospective facilities carefully. Many nursing homes are little more than unsafe institutions where the elderly and dying are shut out of sight. Hazards of poor institutions include unclean facilities with no safety modifications, poorly trained and overworked staff, and inadequate care. In a 2003 report by AARP, more than one-third (36.2 percent) of nursing homes in the United States did not meet federal health and safety standards, and nearly one-third (30.5 percent) were deficient in the quality of care they offered.

In the 2004 National Nursing Home Survey, researchers concluded that the low standards of these facilities may be partly due to profit motives. About 62 percent of nursing homes are privately owned and operated. Because the owners want to make a profit, they may try to keep costs as low as possible, sometimes by providing inadequate care.

ASSISTED LIVING CENTERS

Assisted living centers are the fastest growing residential services available for older adults. Assisted living offers services tailored to those who do not require round-the-clock skilled nursing care but who do need extra help in performing daily tasks.

Usually less expensive than nursing homes, most assisted living centers provide an environment that is more like a home and less like a hospital. These facilities provide housing and care to frail older persons or persons with disabilities while maintaining an emphasis on independence and privacy.

Most assisted living centers offer private rooms or apartments along with large common areas for activities and meals. A staff is on call 24 hours a day to help with the activities of daily living such as bathing, dressing, and getting to meals, as well as housekeeping and laundry. Other services offered at most facilities are medication reminders and assistance in taking medications, transportation, security, health monitoring, social activities, and recreation. Many centers offer graduated levels of care, from transportation and social activities to full-time, skilled nursing. Quality facilities also offer care management—an ongoing assessment and reevaluation of the medical, functional, emotional and social needs of the resident.

The primary goal of assisted living is to allow the resident to live with as much independence and autonomy as possible while minimizing the risks associated with that independence. For instance, if a resident enjoys cooking but forgets to turn off the stove, the staff can provide supervision and reminders that allow the resident to enjoy that activity without endangering anyone.

ADULT DAY CARE

Adult day care centers, sometimes called adult day services, provide an alternative to residential care for the elderly. Adult day care facilities provide health and therapeutic care, as well as social activities, for physically and cognitively impaired older adults. At the same time, they offer family caregivers a break, or respite, from full-time care of aging parents or grandparents. The number of adult day care centers in the United States grew from 300 in 1978 to 2,100 in the 1980s. In 2002, there were more than 4,000 adult day care centers in the United States, according to the National Adult Day Services Association (NADSA). According to NADSA, the rapid increase in adult day care centers is due partly to an increased emphasis on home- and community-based care.

Adult day care centers offer supervised care for people with chronic illnesses, traumatic brain injuries, developmental disabilities, and other problems that interfere with their ability to care for themselves but who live in their own homes or with a relative. Adult day care centers originated as a way of providing a break to family caregivers. These facilities continue to offer a respite for family caregivers, especially those who work or who need some time away from their loved one to complete projects, socialize, or simply take some time for themselves.

Adult day care centers generally fall into three categories:

- Social care, which offers social activities, meals, recreation, and some health-related services;

- Health care, which provides health, social, and therapeutic service for those with severe medical problems and who might otherwise need nursing home care; or

- Alzheimer's-specific adult day care, which serves only persons with Alzheimer's disease or related dementia.

Care is usually provided during weekdays and working hours, which allows family caregivers to continue working even when an elderly parent needs 24-hour care. Most adult day care centers do not provide services on weekends, although some, especially those with religious affiliations, may offer half-day services on Sundays. The range of services provided often includes personal care, transportation, meals, health screening and monitoring, educational programs, counseling, and rehabilitative services. Skilled nursing services are available at most sites, as is transportation. Some centers offer transportation at no extra cost, while others charge by the trip or number of miles.

When choosing an adult day care facility, caregivers should ask if the facility staff performs a needs assessment to determine the person's range of abilities and needs and develops an individualized treatment plan for each participant. The facility should be inspected for cleanliness and safety features. The range of activities and services offered should be clearly explained by the staff. Caregivers and the elderly patient should then determine if the adult day care center meets their needs.

A FAMILY MEMBER WITH ALZHEIMER'S

Alzheimer's disease is a progressive, degenerative brain disorder. People with Alzheimer's experience memory loss, disorientation, changes in behavior, and loss of thinking abilities. As Alzheimer's disease progresses, they gradually lose the ability to speak and move. Alzheimer's disease is most common in people over 65, although it can affect persons of any age. As people live longer, the prevalence of Alzheimer's disease is increasing. The 2009 World Alzheimer Report, released by Alzheimer's Disease International, a nonprofit federation of 71 national Alzheimer organizations, estimates that the global prevalence of dementia, predicted to be more than 35 million in 2010, will almost double every 20 years to 65.7 million in 2030 and 115.4 million in 2050.

Although no cure for Alzheimer's disease exists, some drugs can help control symptoms. People with Alzheimer's live an average of eight years after being diagnosed; some may live for as many as 20 years. The financial and emotional costs of the disease are untold. The stresses on families, children, and other caregivers are so great that Alzheimer's is often called the "family disease." The chronic stress of watching a loved one slowly decline in mental and physical functioning causes problems for everyone in the person's family and caregiving network.

A person with Alzheimer's may be unable to respond to affection and caring, making it difficult for family members to provide compassionate and consistent care. Instead of being thankful for help provided by children or other caregivers, some people with Alzheimer's disease become verbally abusive, violent, and dangerous to themselves and others. During the early stages of the disease, the person may seem perfectly all right one moment and disoriented a few moments later. Such behavior can be disconcerting to family members, for the elderly parent may appear to be getting better and then worse when, in fact, this is just a normal progression of the disease.

As Alzheimer's progresses, the stress on family members increases. A treatment program for anyone with Alzheimer's disease should take into consideration the needs of the family. Training and support groups can help family members learn how to control unwanted behaviors, improve communication, and keep the person with Alzheimer's—as well as themselves—safe. The Family Caregiver Alliance recommends that caregivers prepare themselves in specific ways for each stage of the disease. During the first stage, the emphasis should be on education, emotional support, and planning for the future.

Family members who are caring for the parent with Alzheimer's need the emotional support of other family members, friends, and other sources. Counseling and support groups can help caregivers deal with the emotional issues that arise as the parent progressively declines. The person's role in the family changes as a result of the disease, which can bring up many issues in the family. An Alzheimer's patient will gradually lose the ability to perform tasks ranging from maintaining household finances to remembering to take out the trash. Families should consult a lawyer to help them to ensure that the elderly parent is cared for by family members and that his or her finances remain in trusted hands.

In middle-stage Alzheimer's, the patient needs full-time supervision and family members need to find options for respite, in or out of the home. Safety becomes paramount, both for the person with Alzheimer's and for caregivers. An occupational therapist can offer advice about home modification and devices that can make the home safer. Family members must act as the person's medical care spokesperson, communicating with physicians and other healthcare providers and making decisions about which course of medical care to pursue. Some families may find this an appropriate time to investigate options other than in-home care.

As Alzheimer's progresses to late-stage, caregivers are faced with the end of their parent's life. If the person is still living at home or with a family, consideration should be given to placement in a skilled nursing facility. Hospice services, which are designed to support individuals at the end of life, may help to ease the burden on family members and provide dignified death. Hospice services include support groups, visiting nurses, pain management, and home care. These services are arranged through a physician, usually when the physician recognizes that the person is six months or less from the end of life.

PAYING THE BILLS

As people age, health-care costs increase and incomes go down. Findings from the 2009 MetLife Market Survey of Nursing Home and Home Care Costs show that the average daily cost of a private room in a nursing home is $219—about $6,500 a month or more than $79,000 a year. A companion survey of assisted living facilities, also performed by MetLife researchers, showed that the average monthly cost of care in an assisted living facility was $3,131 in 2009, or $37,572 annually. The price of adult day care, according to the National Adult Day Services Association, averages $67 a day, which can add up to more than $24,000 annually. The Alzheimer's Association reports that 70 percent of Alzheimer's patients live at home, where three-fourths of their care is provided by family and friends.

These expenses stand in stark contrast to the declining incomes of many elderly family members. Data from the U.S. Census Bureau show that in 2008, 9.7 percent of people age 65 and over lived below the federal poverty level of $10,400 per year for a single person. The percentage of people in poverty increases as they enter the middle-old and oldest-old groups. Gender also affects the likelihood that a person will live out their last years in poverty. American Community Survey

2008 data show that of people 65 and older, 7.8 percent of men and 11.9 percent of women were living below the poverty level.

Ethnicity and race are factors in the probability that an older person lives in poverty. Among people 65 and older, almost 25 percent of African Americans, 21 percent of Hispanic Americans, and 10.6 percent of Asian Americans age 65 and older were living in poverty in 2008. During that same year, fewer than 11 percent of white Americans older than 65 years of age were living in poverty.

Many people assume, wrongly, that Medicare and standard health insurance plans will cover the costs associated with in-home care, nursing homes, or assisted living centers. Unfortunately, this is not usually the case. The Family Caregiver Alliance suggests that families review their insurance coverage and investigate public and private sources of healthcare financing. When considering a facility, families should investigate exactly what costs are included in the standard monthly or daily charge, and which services—transportation, nursing care, meals, medications, laundry—will involve additional charges. Several sources of funding for long-term care exist:

- **Long-term care** health insurance plans can help people protect personal assets and inheritance while offering more options in the choice of care environments. Federal health legislation enacted in 2000 helped to make private long-term insurance an option in paying for long-term care costs without loss of personal savings, dignity, or choice. For a person age 50, the average annual premium for a long-term care policy is $1,230; at age 65, it is about $3,290; at 79, it is about $4,110.

- **Medicare** is a federal health insurance program for people 65 and over and certain disabled people under 65. Long-term care is not covered by Medicare nor are assisted living costs. Some short-term services such as physical therapy are paid for by Medicare. Nursing facility coverage is extremely limited.

- **Medicaid** is a federal-state program that provides health-care assistance to low-income people. Medicaid is the major payer for nursing home services. In some states, it also offers limited coverage of assisted living services and adult day care. To qualify for Medicaid, the person needing care must prove that his or her financial resources have been depleted. If the person is married, states allow the at-home spouse to retain enough from the couple's income to bring the at-home spouse's income to 150 percent of the federal poverty level for a two-person household.

- The Department of Veterans Affairs, the government agency that offers benefits and services to people who have served in the armed forces, provides care to veterans who need nursing care, both in its own facilities and through contracts with community nursing homes. All veterans qualify for these services.

ELDERLY FAMILY MEMBERS MOVING IN

While nursing homes, day care, home nursing, assisted living, and other community care services are important resources for persons in late adulthood, the most important resource an elderly person can have is a responsible and caring family. Most elderly people prefer to remain in their own homes, where they can maintain independence and privacy. Likewise, most adults prefer to live in separate homes from their parents. Both parents and grown children, if given a choice, would live close enough so that visiting is easy while maintaining separate households. Community support programs such as "Meals on Wheels," which offers free meals to homebound seniors, can help seniors to remain in their own homes.

As the care needs of an elderly family member increase, families often relocate the person into the adult child's home. Data from the U.S. census show that in *1998*, about one out of 10 men and one out of five women age 65 years and older were living in the homes of their adult children.

The decision for an elderly parent to move into an adult child's home requires careful consideration of the needs of the parent, the adult child, and the other family members. Providing extensive care for someone with severe medical, functional, and cognitive problems can cause extreme stress and hardship for caregivers. Family members should openly discuss all possible options for care of the elderly parent, the role each person will play in the transition, changes in lifestyle, management of finances, and safety modifications to the home.

TEENS SPEAK

My Grandfather Lives With Us

My grandfather moved in with us about two years ago, when I was 15. Before that, I saw him once or twice a year at his home in Georgia. The last time was at my sister's wedding. He danced the whole night. So when, on a windy mid-February Chicago day two months after the wedding, an old man in a wheelchair arrived at our house, it was hard to believe that it was my grandfather. He had suffered a stroke and couldn't use his right hand or leg. I felt embarrassed for him on that first night as I watched my mother cut his meat into small pieces so he could eat it.

I helped my dad build wheelchair ramps and install bars in the bathrooms and hallways so my grandfather could get around the house. He couldn't go upstairs because of the wheelchair, so I had to move out of my room on the first floor. He was really grumpy at first. He complained about my music, my hairstyle, my clothes, and my friends.

I'll confess, I was angry. After all, I had done everything I could to make him feel at home, even given up my room. And all he could do was complain. But one evening when I was watching television and Granddad was sitting in his wheelchair, playing a solitary game of checkers, he asked me to give him the remote control. I thought he was going to change the channel, but instead, he turned the television off and asked if I had time to talk. I couldn't think of any excuses to get away. He told me he was sorry for making life harder for my family and that he was thankful for all we were doing for him. He said he had a lot of stories he would like to tell before he died, and he asked me if I would help him write them down.

That was how I started getting to know my grandfather. About three times a week, we sit down with a tape recorder and a pen and paper, and I write and ask him questions about his life. I never knew what an interesting life he had led. He told me about growing up on a farm in northern Minnesota, meeting my grandmother, fighting in Vietnam, and many other things I never knew about him. He may not be able to do many of the things he used to do anymore, but I've learned a lot about him and the rest of my family, including things my mother never knew.

When an elderly family member moves into an adult child's home, traditional roles change. The elderly parent may no longer be able to act as a parent—making decisions, giving direction and guidance, and determining the best choices for family members. The family's children may need to assist with household responsibilities and with care of the grandparent. Agreements should be developed about lifestyle issues such as bedtimes and nap times, food choices at mealtimes, and noise levels in the house.

Although the integration of an elderly parent into an adult child's home may be difficult and challenging, many adult children find it rewarding to be able to give support and care to their parents. For grandchildren, living with a grandparent can be a chance to learn about family history and family connectedness.

Q & A

Question: How can I deal with my grandparents' divorce?

Answer: Your divorcing grandparents need your support more than ever. Divorce is difficult for any couple, but for those over 60, divorce can be devastating. Late-life divorce can negatively affect the relations between parents and young adult children. In 1994, sociologist W. S. Aquilino studied 3,281 young adults whose parents divorced late in life. Aquilino found a marked decrease in the quality of parent-child relations. You may need to make an extra effort to maintain contact with both of your grandparents. Remember, they're divorcing each other, not you. Set aside some time to spend with each of them. Ask your grandparents questions about their lives. You might be surprised by what you find.

Late adulthood is often a time of transition from independence to physical dependence. These changes can be difficult for the elderly family member to accept. Nursing homes, assisted living facilities, and adult day care services offer care ranging from help with personal tasks to skilled nursing care.

When elderly parents move into their adult children's homes, the parent, the adult child, and other family members are all affected. Caregiving can be stressful, but it can also be rewarding.

See also: Day Care; Death in the Family; Family, The New; Family, The Traditional; Financial Management, Marital; Marriage and Family, Changes in; Religion and the Family

FURTHER READING

Berman, Raeann, and Bernard Shulman. *Caring for Your Aging Parents: An Emotional Guide to Nurturing Your Loved Ones while Taking Care of Yourself.* Naperville, Ill.: Sourcebooks Inc., 2009.

Kind, Viki. *The Caregiver's Path to Compassionate Decision Making: Making Choices for Those Who Can't.* Austin, Tex.: Greenleaf Book Group LLC, 2010.

Loverde, Joy. *Eldercare Planner: Where to Start, Which Questions to Ask, and How to Find Help.* New York: Crown Publishing Group, 2009.

■ ETHNICITY AND EXPECTATIONS

Preconceived notions, of society in general and educators in particular, that are based on peoples' race, the country their family originally came from, their cultural heritage, or other factors related to one's ethnic background. Society often tries to predict how successful a person will be based solely on generalizations about a larger group with whom that person is identified, and educators, employers, and others will sometimes treat people of certain ethnic backgrounds differently as a result.

Most of the time, it is plainly unfair to judge a person based only on ethnicity, because each person is different and should be judged on individual accomplishments, skills, and talents. However, such **bias** or prejudice is a fact of life, and it can help to understand where it comes from and ways to deal with it.

CREATING CATEGORIES

Most everyone can agree that a **stereotype** is a bad thing, because it causes people to prejudge someone based only on factors such as

DID YOU KNOW?

Even Positive Stereotypes Can Be Harmful

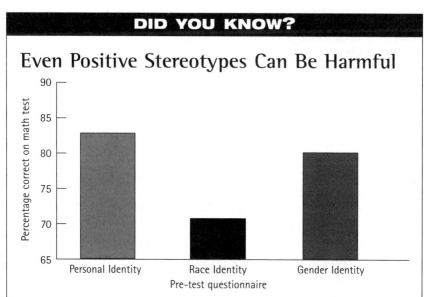

Stereotypes affect performance, and in this case, math scores. A group of Asian American women were all given the same math test. However, the women were given three different pre-test questionnaires, each focusing on one of three aspects of the women's identity. For those women whose questionnaires had focused on their personal identity or on their gender, they achieved similar scores, above the 80 percentile. However, when the pre-test questionnaire focused on racial identity—even though that stereotype is based on Asian women's performing better in math—those women did poorly. Researchers say that any focus on ethnicity, even in a positive way, puts additional pressure on test-takers and makes it difficult to concentrate.

Source: "Cognitive Daily" blog at scienceblogs.com (posted December 16, 2005), at http://scienceblogs.com/cognitivedaily/2005/12/the_negative_impact_of_positiv.php.

race, religion, where a person comes from, what he or she looks like, and other largely superficial factors. Stereotypes can be rooted in real ugliness, sometimes not only keeping prejudices of the past alive but also sustaining unfair categories for the present and future.

Why do stereotypes exist? Simply because they provide one way for people to try to make sense of the world: by creating categories—often based on misconceptions, past experience, and simple ignorance—and putting people into them. The world is a much easier place to understand if you can judge someone just by looking at his or her skin color, gender, style of dress, behavior, even body type—and draw conclusions, both positive and negative, about them. As a result, many people reach conclusions that are largely inaccurate and potentially damaging. It extends to a person's ethnic background: For example, presupposing that an Asian student will be good at math, even though he may be more interested in art and music, is an unwanted expectation that might prevent that student from pursuing his dreams.

Especially for children and teenagers, the result of stereotyping can be particularly damaging. It can change the way parents, teachers, and others, both adults and peers, think of young students. Judging people can change the way people expect them to perform in school and in life. As a result, a boy or girl might be pushed in a direction that is wrong for him or her, simply because of the way that person looks or where he or she comes from. Categories are created, and people are forced into those categories, which can be very difficult for a person who may not belong there. Moreover, students can start to believe that the categories fit.

TEENS SPEAK

What Am I?

My mom grew up in Brooklyn, in a Jewish neighborhood. My grandfather, her dad, was African American. My grandmother, her mom, was both Jewish and Polish. My dad was born in Jamaica—the country, not the neighborhood of Queens in New York—and immigrated to America with his parents in 1965, when he was two years old. My grandmother and grandfather on my dad's side were killed in a car accident three years after arriving in Philadelphia, and my dad was adopted and raised by a Greek couple who lived next door and were close friends of the family.

My mom, who is half-black, is light-skinned and considered herself Jewish, but as a teenager she converted to Islam. My father is dark-skinned and Roman Catholic. I have been brought up with knowledge of all three religions, but I find myself drawn to Buddhism. We still eat latkes at Hanukkah, and my dad loves Greek treats around the holidays, because it always reminds him of his childhood in Philadelphia.

I like to play chess and hockey and basketball. My older brother is a rapper; my sister is learning ballet. In the summer we all love ice cream and going to concerts in the park.

I hate that people might look at me and think, just by looking at me, that they know who or what I am. Tell me: What am I?

HOW DIFFERENT ARE WE?

Many studies have examined and broken down academic performance by ethnicity and found trends: Some did better than others on tests in school. Originally, researchers focused on **genetics** as an explanation for performance, suggesting that some groups were inherently, or naturally, more gifted intellectually than others. However, most studies have focused on a wide range of other factors that can explain the differences.

For example, different cultures put a different emphasis on success in school, partly because they had been assigned different tasks in society based on ethnicity—as farmhands, for example, or factory workers—and so measured success in different ways. Generations later, a **ripple effect** is still felt, as parents pass along many of the lessons they were taught, which were the same that their parents were taught.

Language differences also can play a big role: If someone is raised in a household in which a language other than English is spoken, it can make it much more difficult for that student to understand the teacher in a classroom. Test scores might be lower as a result, but it would be unfair and inaccurate to say that is because the student is not as smart as his or her classmates. This would be a misconception and an unfair judgment based on an ethnic difference.

Fact Or Fiction?

People of different ethnicities are significantly different, right down to their genes.

The Facts: As early as the 15th century, and continuing through the 20th century, the concept of "race" was based on the belief that the human species can be divided up by physical traits—skin color, hair texture, facial features—and that those traits were based on genetic differences. However, modern scientists have debunked most of that thinking, agreeing that in reality there are no distinct "races"—just one human race. In the 1970s, geneticists found that only a very small proportion (6 percent or less) of human genetic variability occurs. The notion of "ethnicity" has generally replaced the notion of "race," grouping people based on language, customs, and other factors. Genetically, we are all mostly the same.

THE ROLE OF EXPECTATIONS

Evidence shows that expectations themselves help to keep stereotypes going. For instance, in a study outlined in the *Journal of School Psychology* in June 2008, two psychology professors looked at nearly 2,000 elementary age students in 83 classrooms in which the students said teachers treated the better students much differently than the students who scored less well on tests. The classrooms had a mixture of students from various ethnic backgrounds.

The researchers found that the teachers expected significantly more from students with a European or Asian ethnic background than they did from African-American or Latino students—even among students with similar records of achievement in the past. It seemed to confirm that ethnicity affects what people expect from young people, and it is easy to see how that can affect those students and how they perceive themselves, their strengths and weaknesses, and their chances for success.

Q & A

Question: What does "ethnicity" mean, literally?

Answer: According to the *American Heritage New Dictionary of Cultural Literacy,* Third Edition, *ethnicity* is defined as "identity with or membership in a particular racial, national, or cultural group and observance of that group's customs, beliefs, and language." Whether ethnicity affects your expectations of people is up to you.

WHAT YOU CAN DO

Life is not always fair—we all know that to be true. It is a simple fact that some people, even well-meaning adults, mistakenly lump people together for the wrong reasons and have different expectations based on something other than a person's abilities.

So what can you do? The first step is to be honest about your concerns and talk with your family, teachers, and guidance counselors about your goals and interests. Most people fall back on categories before they know a person well, but they are more than willing to adjust these attitudes based on what they learn about an individual. Therefore, make sure the adults around you know your interests. If you enjoy certain subjects, say so—and get involved with activities connected to them. Read books on your favorite subjects, not just the ones on your class reading lists.

Also, although you should get advice and guidance when you need it, make sure you do not let people put you into a category that simply does not feel comfortable. Be yourself, rather than being something people think you should be. You might help change not only expectations about you but also change the way your teachers will treat the next class to come along.

See also: Families, Blended; Families, Racially Mixed; Family Traditions; Marriage and Family, Changes in; Religion and the Family.

FURTHER READING

Cornell, Stephen E. *Ethnicity and Race: Making Identities in a Changing World.* Newbury Park, Calif.: Pine Forge Press, 2006.
Waters, Mary C. *Ethnic Options: Choosing Identity in America.* Berkeley: University of California Press, 1990.

▮ FAMILIES, BLENDED

A family created when a divorced or widowed person marries someone who may or may not have been married before. One or both spouses may bring children from a previous marriage to the new union. Blended families are also called **reconstituted families** or **stepfamilies.**

REMARRIAGES

About half of all Americans have been or will be in a blended family at some time during their lives. In 1998, the last year in which the Census Bureau collected data on remarriages, almost half of all new marriages—46 percent—were remarriages for the husband, wife, or both. Children from previous marriages are often brought to the new relationship. Data from the 2000 census show that in that year, an estimated 3.2 million children were living with a stepparent. More than one-third of all children in the United States will live in a blended family before they reach the age of 18.

Census Bureau data of 2001 indicate that about two-thirds of people who divorce each year eventually remarry. Most remarriages occur within a few years of divorce. The median interval between divorce and remarriage is three years for women and four and one-half years for men. Whether a divorced person remarries, and how quickly, is influenced by ethnic background. The rate of remarriage is highest for whites, who also remarry most quickly. Latinos are slower to remarry, while African Americans are less likely to remarry at all. In 1998, 44 percent of white women had remarried within three years of a divorce, while 20 percent of African-American women and 23 percent of Latina women had remarried. The lower rates of remarriage among African-American women may be partly due to the lack of availability of single, economically stable African-American men.

Remarriages are slightly more likely to end in divorce than first marriages, which means that about half of the children who experience one parental divorce will experience a second. The chance that a remarriage will end in divorce is greater when one or both spouses have children from previous relationships. In "Labor Market and Socioeconomic Effects on Marital Stability," a 1995 study of the effects of economic factors on marriages that dissolved between the mid-1960s and the mid-1980s, sociologists Jessie Tzeng and Robert Mare found that couples in which the woman is remarried are almost twice as likely to divorce as couples in which the man is the remarried partner. They hypothesized that this may be partly due to the greater likelihood that a woman who remarries will bring children to the relationship. Tzeng and Mare noted that the rate of divorce is 50 percent higher in marriages in which children are present than in those in which there are no children from previous marriages.

Fact Or Fiction?

Blended families are just like other families.

The Facts: Expecting a blended family to function exactly like a biological family can lead to surprise, disappointment, and bewilderment. Parents and children can both play into this dynamic. Stepparents, having been married previously, may expect that they will quickly jump into their new parenting role, only to be surprised when stepchildren don't react to them as they do to their biological parents. Children may feel jealous of their biological parent's new spouse. Teens are likely to reject any attempt by the stepparent to act like a parent. Blended families do better when family members recognize that relationships between the individuals in blended families differ from those in biological families. Time is required to build a sense of family. The remarriage of a parent is usually accompanied by a very unstable period, which may last for as long as five to seven years. In most blended families, restabilization occurs after five years, with relationship patterns becoming more like those in non-divorced families. Blended families must create flexible family boundaries to navigate an often-complex network of custodial and noncustodial parents and extended family members. Stepparents should also recognize that they cannot replace a biological parent and may need to create their own nontraditional parenting role.

Women continue to be more likely to be the custodial parent from a previous marriage. Census Bureau data show that in 2008, 73 percent of the 19.3 million custodial parents in the United States were women.

Children's adjustment to a parent's remarriage is affected by their age, according to the American Psychological Association (APA). In a nine-year longitudinal study funded by the National Institute of Child Health and Human Development, published in the *Journal of Family Psychology*, James Bray, a researcher and clinician at the department of family medicine at Baylor College of Medicine, found that adjustment to parental remarriage seems to be most difficult for children ages 10 to 14.

Bray's results showed that before age 10, children are generally more accepting of a new adult in the family, especially if the adult is a positive influence. Children ages 10 to 14 may have had more difficulty adjusting to a parent's remarriage, partly because they are going through the emotional and physiological changes of adolescence, forming their own identities, and separating from their families. At the same time that the new blended family is trying to establish close ties, young teens are testing their independence. Still, as they experiment with issues of identity and independence, they need a stable family framework to provide continuity. Teens age 15 and older in Bray's sample fared better, in part, because they may need less parenting and have less investment in stepfamily life.

THE PERCEPTION OF PLAYING FAVORITES

Blended families involve complicated networks of relationship. A child may have relationships with a custodial mother, a noncustodial father, a stepfather, two sets of biological grandparents, stepgrandparents, siblings, and step-siblings. Half of all women who remarry will bear a child with the new spouse, adding yet another layer of complexity to family relationships. In this complex network of relationships, it is all too easy for the parent, the new spouse, and the children to appear to favor one child over another.

Several studies, including Bray's, also found that children may resist the new stepparent's entry into the family and perceive him or her as intruding into their relationship with the custodial parent or cutting off their relationship with the noncustodial parent. They may have been hoping that their parents will get back together; a parent's remarriage forces them to face the reality that their parents' marriage is over.

Tensions can create competition between the new spouse and the partner's children. Children may feel jealous of the time and attention their parent is giving to the new spouse. In turn, the new spouse may resent the time and attention the parent gives to stepchildren. Parents may feel guilty about the emotional turmoil and upheaval that children experienced at the ending of their former marriage and try to make up for it by overindulging the child. Any of these or similar situations can result in the perception of playing favorites.

Q & A

Question: How can I get along with my new stepmother?

Answer: Your new stepmother probably feels about as nervous about your relationship as you do. Ask her if you can do something together that you both enjoy. It might be taking a walk, getting an ice cream cone, or taking a drive. Just be sure that it's a setting where you'll have time to talk with her without interruptions. You may feel angry and resentful toward your stepmother; that's okay. You don't have to love her right now. Treat her with respect and let her know that you expect her to do the same for you. Remember that you don't have to choose between your biological mother and your stepmother. You can develop a special, separate relationship with each of them. You have two adult women in your life who can mentor you and help you face life's challenges.

GETTING ALONG: ISSUES FOR STEPCHILDREN

For most children, the remarriage of a parent means the introduction of not only another adult into their home but also new siblings. Children may suddenly be required to share a bedroom that was once their personal domain. **Sibling rivalry**—the competition between brothers and sisters for their parents' attention, approval, and affection—may be magnified in stepfamilies.

TEENS SPEAK

I Was Furious About Having a New Stepsister

Three years after my dad and mom divorced, he started dating Anna, who is now my stepmom. I liked Anna, but it was hard to think that my dad was dating another woman besides my mom. But when, about a year later, he told me that he and Anna were getting married and that she and her daughter Michelle were going to move into our house, I was furious.

It was the only house I had ever lived in. Dad and I had stayed there after my parents' divorce. I felt like the house was the only thing left of my parents' marriage. Having Anna in my house was going to be bad enough, but being required to share my space with Michelle was even worse. To me, it was simple: Michelle was an invader in my space. I stayed angry for a long time after the wedding. I made no excuses. I hated Michelle, and I told her so to her face. She told me the same thing. We fought about dumb things like whose turn it was to clean up after dinner. You might as well have declared war than have the two of us in the same room with one television. Whoever had the remote control would mastermind the channels while the other complained noisily about how lousy the show was. One day I finally got fed up and unplugged the television. Dad and Anna had to stop us before we hurt each other.

Something happened that night. Michelle and I were both crying and angry. I remember looking at her and realizing that she felt just as hurt and scared and disappointed as I did about our parents' divorcing and remarrying. I knew that no matter how miserable I made life for Michelle, she and Anna were staying. They were the family that I had, and I could accept that or fight it and make life miserable for all of us.

It's been six years now since Michelle and Anna moved in. I'll be leaving for college in the fall. And you know what? I'm going to miss her. We may not be biological sisters, but I'm glad to have her as my stepsister. After all, she knows what it's like to live through your parents' divorce and remarriage.

The first reactions of step-siblings to each other do not always predict the future. Children can seem distant, jealous, and uncertain of each other at first, then develop a relationship of trust and loyalty. Older step-siblings may become protective of younger step-siblings, who, in turn, may idolize older siblings. Relationships between biological siblings may be more contentious than between step-siblings, especially during the teenage years, according to psychologist E. Mavis Hetherington. She suggests that the difference may be due to a lack of a clear definition of step-sibling roles. Also step-siblings may not be as closely involved in each other's lives as biological siblings, which leads to less conflict.

When a remarried woman gives birth, the effect on siblings and step-siblings appears to be positive. Many couples report that having a baby improves step-sibling relationships. In *Coping with Divorce, Single Parenting, and Remarriage: A Risk and Resiliency Perspective,* Hetherington and colleagues present the results of "The Dynamics of Parental Remarriage," a study that found no children responded negatively to the birth of a new step-sibling. Hetherington and her colleagues suggest that the arrival of a new baby can help the two groups of children form a bond.

FINANCES: YOUR MONEY, MY MONEY

Finances, an issue in many marriages, can be an especially hot topic for remarried couples. A divorced and remarried father may need to pay child support to his ex-wife, maintain the new household, and support his new partner's children. A divorced and remarried mother may contribute her earnings to the household, receive child support from her ex-husband, and help support her new partner's children.

In 1983, psychologist Barbara Fishman published "The Economic Behavior of Stepfamilies," a study of financial arrangements in blended families. Her widely cited study is still used by sociologists, demographers, psychologists, and other researchers. Fishman interviewed 100 people who lived in 16 middle-class blended families. She asked detailed questions about economic decisions within the families. Fishman found two common economic patterns used by blended families, which she called the **common-pot method** and the **two-pot method**.

Couples who use the common-pot approach pool their earnings in a joint account. Those earnings may include income from employment, child support, and other sources. The family distributes resources according to the needs of each family member, not according to biological relationship. For instance, the biological child of one parent may be attending college, which puts a strain on the entire family's resources. If the family uses the common-pot approach, the cost of the child's college education comes out of the shared household resources. In reality, it may mean that the child's stepmother may put off buying items such as a new car until the child finishes college.

The couples in Fishman's study who used the two-pot method contribute an agreed-upon amount to household maintenance but keep his or her own resources for personal use or to support biological children. Pooled resources are used to pay fixed expenses such as a mortgage, gas, and electricity. The children, however, are supported by their biological parents. In the example used above, the college expenses of the father's biological child would be his responsibility and the stepmother would be free to invest her personal resources in the new car.

Among the couples in Fishman's study, the two-pot method encouraged biologically related family members to maintain loyalties and personal autonomy, while the common-pot approach helped to unify the blended family. She concluded that the financial commitment that family members make appears to reflect their commitment and the strength of interpersonal bonds in the blended family. Financial commitment to a new spouse may be slow to develop, and a financial commitment to a new spouse's children may develop even more slowly, if at all.

WHO GIVES UP THE HOUSE?

Most people who remarry face the difficult decision of who will leave an established household. In general, remarrying couples have three options: she and her children (if any) move in with him, he and his children (if any) move in with her, or they both relocate to a new home. Employment, finances, and the roominess of the living space are primary factors in deciding who gives up the house.

According to the American Psychological Association, couples who choose the third option—relocating to a new house—are taking an important step toward building a unified blended family. In contrast to the tensions that may develop when one partner and children move into the other's space, moving into a new home allows both partners and their children to start fresh.

However, it may not be financially feasible for the new couple to buy a new home. If they stay in one partner's house, they have to modify established routines. Couples should carefully discuss available options with their children, especially preteens and teens.

NEW SCHOOL?

Teens who experience the remarriage of their custodial parent are also likely to change residences, and with that change may come a change in schools. Changing schools is a stressful event for anyone, but when combined with the stresses of adjusting to a blended family, it may be especially difficult. Even if the move is only to a different section of town, moving to a new school means less interaction with friends, familiar places, and routines.

For children of divorced parents, the disruptive effect of moving to a new school may be very strong. In the November 2002 issue of the *Journal of Marriage and the Family,* Kathleen Rodgers and Hilary Rose, researchers from Washington State University, demonstrated that the ability of teens to adjust to divorce—which they call adolescent resiliency—is strongly affected by the support they receive at school. The researchers studied 2,011 teens who lived in intact families, blended families, and single-parent families. The researchers evaluated the teens' level of parental support and nonfamily support and asked about risk-taking behaviors such as the use of alcohol or tobacco. While parental support and monitoring helped to decrease teens' self-destructive behaviors, nonfamily support was at least equally as important. Significantly, of all the nonfamily factors that the researchers examined, attachment to school had the greatest effect on a teen's mental well-being.

Teens *can* and do cope with the changes that a move to a new school brings. Attending a new school does not necessarily mean losing friendships. Visits with friends from the old school can help to ease the transition. Teens may feel embarrassed about the divorce and remarriage of their parents, but there is no reason for them to feel this way. It's almost a given that many other teens at the school also come from blended families.

The challenge of making friends at the new school is a big concern for many teens. At a new school, teens may have to go out of their way to introduce themselves to others. Indicators of shared interest are good places to start conversations. Getting involved in sports and other extracurricular activities can also help teens make new friends and adapt to a new school.

NEW STATE?

A parent's remarriage may mean that teens must relocate to a new state, far from friends, the noncustodial parent, and other family members. Moving far away from familiar people and places may bring up feelings of anxiety, sadness, and anger for all family members. Teens and preteens may resist moving away from a familiar home. This resistance is not mere stubbornness. According to the *American Psychological Association,* such resistance often reflects the important developmental work that they are doing in their lives. One aspect of this developmental work is learning how to form long-term relationships, including romantic ones. The prospect of moving seems to tear apart the ties that they have carefully been forming. Having to move because a parent remarries is also a harsh reminder that the teen is not yet an independent adult. When a parent's remarriage is accompanied by a move, the changes can seem overwhelming.

Parents and children of all ages can work together to make the move to a new state the first step toward creating a unified new blended family. According to TeenGrowth.com, a physician-reviewed Web site for teens, teens adapt better to a family relocation when they are involved in the move from the start. Many teens are adept internet users and can cybersurf to research the new community. Anxiety about the move may be lessened if the family visits the new home and becomes familiar with the new community and its resources.

Before the move, parents can schedule frequent family meetings to talk about the upcoming relocation and the changes it will bring for each member of the family. Each person should have a chance to express his or her feelings without criticism.

After the move, telephone calls, e-mails, letters, and visits from friends at the old school can help family members make the transition smoother. For some older teens—seniors in high school, for example— the best alternative might be to stay behind with a trusted family friend or relative for a year.

A blended family is created when a divorced or widowed person marries another person who may or may not have been married before. About half of all Americans have been or will be in a blended family at some time during their lives. Because children most often live with their mothers after divorce, most blended families include a biological mother, her children, and a stepfather. In this complex network of relationship, tensions and anger can erupt between family members. Couples who pool financial resources tend to display greater commitment. When parents remarry, teens and other family members may need to move. While these changes can be difficult, teens who actively participate in the move and maintain contact with their established lives, can eventually adjust.

See also: Arguments and the Family; Divorce and Families; Families, Divided; Families, Racially Mixed; Family, The New; Family, The Traditional; Financial Management, Marital; Marriage and Family, Changes in; Single-Parent Families; Stepparents

FURTHER READING
Deal, Ron. *The Smart Stepfamily: Seven Steps to a Healthy Family.* Bloomington, Minn.: Bethany House Publishers, 2006.

■ FAMILIES, DIVIDED

Conflict between family members that leads to short or long-term alienation of family members from each other is known as estrangement.

Conflicts may involve only two individuals, or family members may "take sides." Estrangement may last for days, weeks, years, or generations. Often, however, long-lasting divisions in families can be avoided or healed.

WHY FAMILIES DIVIDE

Divisions in families arise as a result of interpersonal conflict. Although definitions of interpersonal conflict vary, some sociologists define *interpersonal conflict* by focusing on actions—for example, "an interpersonal process that occurs whenever the actions of one person interfere with the actions of another." Others focus on the philosophy behind conflict, defining it as "interactions between persons expressing opposing interests, view, or opinions."

Divisions in families are often the result of intolerance. Family members may disapprove of each other's lifestyle choices, choice of mate, religious preferences, or educational choices, to name a few topics of frequent conflict. The decision to marry outside one's religion, race, nationality, or **ethnicity** may lead to long-term feuds between family members. Many families have broken apart when dividing a parent's estate. For instance, two sisters may become estranged over what one feels is the unfair division of their recently-deceased mother's belongings. The conflict may focus on a specific item, such as a cherished heirloom piece of jewelry, but the estrangement may really be about the lifelong dynamics between the sisters. The sister who did not receive the jewelry may feel that it is just another way in which her sister was always preferred by her mother and may overreact with anger, resentment, and estrangement.

Teens and parents may be especially vulnerable to conflict that is bitter and long-lasting. Emotions often run high for both teens and parents. Teens are working to establish their own identities and separate from their family. They are forming their own relationships, asking questions about the purpose of their lives, and forming their own beliefs and value systems, which may be markedly different from those of their parents. They are becoming more independent. Parents may react with fear and anger to teen's normal developmental process and his or her experiments with identity and separation from the family. These efforts may result in a reactive, rather than a responsive, cycle of fighting between the teen and his or her parents. The fight may seem to be about the teen's hairstyle or choice of clothing. In reality, the clothing or hairstyle may symbolize the real source of conflict—the teen's attempt to differentiate from the family, and the parents' resistance to those attempts.

COMPROMISE

Often, conflict can be resolved through **compromise**. In a compromise, both sides agree on a mutually acceptable solution that is not exactly what either wanted but is fair and meets each person's minimum needs. Both get some of their wishes fulfilled, but neither is totally satisfied. For instance, Tony may want to go to an American-style restaurant and Joan may prefer to go to a Chinese restaurant; they could compromise by going to a restaurant that serves both types of food. Compromise involves negotiation, a clearly thought-out approach to solving problems and considering all options. When negotiating a compromise, family members state their positions, exchange information in an objective manner, and work toward an acceptable solution.

NEW ALTERNATIVES

If intolerance is the tool that divides a family, tolerance is the key to mending family ties. Tolerance may start with education or acceptance of the other's beliefs and exploring alternative solutions. In many cases, feuding family members can use **integrative agreements** and accommodation to find creative ways to resolve the problem and restore peace.

In integrative agreements, a solution is found in which both parties can achieve their original goals and aspirations. While difficult to achieve, these types of agreements allow each party to pursue central goals while working within the boundaries of the other person's core goals. For instance, a teen and parent may be at odds about where the teen will go to college. They can start by identifying each other's central goals. The parent's central goal for both may be for the teen to attend a college of high academic standing at a reasonable price. The teen's central goal may be to go to a more expensive school because it has an excellent program in veterinary medicine, which she wants to study. The teen and parent may agree that she will start her studies at an in-state college, where tuition is less, take a part-time job, and then apply for scholarships that will allow her to transfer to the school she wants to attend. Integrative agreements require flexibility and **logrolling**, or making concessions on one issue if the other person will make concessions on another, while still maintaining commitment to central goals.

Fact Or Fiction?

Avoiding fights is the best way to handle disagreements.

The Facts: There are "good" fights and "bad" fights. In good fights, the two people remain respectful of each other, listen carefully, validate the other's feelings, and own their own feelings. In bad fights, the two people go at each other mercilessly, with no restraints. Bad fights also occur when one or both people act manipulatively or lie. "Good" fighting is no easy task. It requires self-discipline, genuine caring about the other person, and self-awareness. It requires the ability to recognize and honestly state one's own feelings. But the potential rewards are great. Conflict, instead of leading to lasting feuds and divisions in families, can instead become a chance for everyone involved to grow closer, learn more about each other, and learn more about themselves. Instead of being something to be avoided at all costs, fighting fair can present a challenge and an opportunity for personal growth.

Caryl Rusbult, professor of psychology at the University of North Carolina at Chapel Hill and colleagues describe an alternative method of handling conflict, which they call accommodation. In accommodation, a person does not respond destructively to another person's destructive actions, but instead reacts in a constructive manner. Constructive responses might be loyalty, which involves optimistically waiting for conditions to improve, defending the partner in the face of criticism, or continuing to show signs of involvement. Another constructive response is to give voice to the issue by discussing it with the partner, changing behavior to solve the problem, or consulting a therapist or friend. Destructive responses might take the form of neglect, in which the offended person withdraws, avoids discussion of the problem, or nags the other person about unrelated issues. Exit is an actively destructive response in which the offended person leaves, threatens to end the relationship, or engages in abusive acts such as yelling or hitting.

According to Rusbult, people who are able to accommodate are usually responding out of **effective preferences**. Effective preferences are the actions people want to take when they focus on broad concerns, such as the long-term consequences of their actions and the implications for others. In contrast, **given preferences** are the actions people want to take when they focus only on short-term, self-centered, immediate reactions to an event. When accommodation does occur, it is likely to set in motion a positive cycle of increased trust and willingness to accommodate.

BEING FAIR AT ALL TIMES

Conflict is an inevitable part of life. When people who know each other closely and intimately fight, conflict can be difficult and devastating. Family members know enough about each other to "fight dirty," whether consciously or unconsciously. When families fight, it is especially important that they fight fair. Experts in conflict resolution offer a few suggestions for fighting fair and accomplishing goals:

- Set a time and place.

- Feuding family members should agree on a neutral place and a time that works for everyone. Launching into a fight unexpectedly makes it more likely that things will escalate.

- Establish ground rules. Ground rules should be established in the beginning. They might include allowing everyone to have their say, no interruptions, a system of signaling the wish to respond, and other principles of fairness.

- Be respectful. When feelings are hurt and anger is high, it is difficult to act respectfully toward another. But it is also the most important time to show respect to the other person. Avoid belittling, criticizing, or making fun of the other person. Blanket statements such as "you always" can lead to more animosity.

- Tackle the problem, not the person. The problem should be clearly defined in concrete terms. Who did what? When did they do it? How does it make the other person feel? Give everyone a chance to describe their feelings using statements that begin with "I." Do not seek to shame, belittle, or punish the other person. Name calling or attacking sensitive issues in a spirit of ill will, hatred, revenge, or contempt—"You are such a slob. Can't you ever pick up after yourself?"—will only deepen the conflict. Define the conflict as a problem to be solved by both people working together, not a war to be won.

■ Communicate clearly. Each person should spend at least as much time listening as talking. Everyone should have a chance to say what they need to without interruption. Restate the other person's position to increase understanding: "So what I hear you saying is that you were frightened when I didn't come home until after 2:00 this morning?" Asking questions can help ensure that listeners understand before they explain their positions.

■ Be creative. What solutions might there be that no one has thought of? Family members should take turns offering ideas for ways to develop or find workable solutions.

■ Write a letter of agreement. Whatever solution is reached, it should be explicitly stated, written down, and shared with all family members.

■ Reassess the agreement in a few weeks or months. How is it working? Does it need to be modified in any way? Does everyone still feel it is fair?

Q & A

Question: My father and I fight constantly about the way I keep my room. We haven't spoken since our last fight two months ago. How can I make peace with my father?

Answer: You might want to start by writing your father a letter in which you tell him about your desire to make peace with him. What do you want to say to him about your room? Is it really the state of your room you're fighting about, or are you two fighting about your ability to choose how to maintain your personal space? You may wish to consult a professional therapist or mediator for help in resolving these issues.

MAINTAINING CIVILITY

Laura Davis, author of *I Thought We'd Never Speak Again,* suggests that reconciliation is an ongoing continuum with a spectrum of possible outcomes. According to Davis, the most desired and most difficult to achieve is a deep and transformative reconciliation in which intimacy is reestablished, past hurts resolved, and family members feel closeness and satisfaction.

For example, one family member may be able to change his or her expectations so that interaction can occur with another family member in a positive and caring manner, whether or not the other person makes significant changes. In the third and most difficult type of resolution, much remains unresolved and ambivalent feelings are still present. Both people "agree to disagree" and establish ground rules that allow them to have a limited but courteous relationship. When they realize that no viable relationship is possible, the only option is to find resolution within themselves.

When violations in families are deep, such as in cases of physical or sexual abuse, or the parties cannot create a workable solution, an atmosphere of mutual civility may be all that is possible. Politeness and respect are integral to any interactions. Davis suggests that family members agree on "terms of engagement," or rules the two parties agree to so they can interact peacefully in limited circumstances. Terms of engagement might include avoiding discussions of certain volatile topics, requests that certain types of jokes or stories not be told, boundaries about touch, discussions about where, when, and how interactions should take place, or conditions under which family members are allowed to visit. In extremely difficult and conflicted situations, families should consider professional mediation.

Divisions in families arise as a result of interpersonal conflict between family members. Disputes over deeply held beliefs or values can lead to long-lasting alienation of family members from each other. Teens and parents may be especially vulnerable to divisive conflict, partly because teens are working to establish their own identities and separate from their family. Parents may react with fear and anger to teens' efforts to gain independence. But conflict does not always have to lead to estrangement. Resolving conflict usually requires effort, compromise, and agreement from all family members. By learning to fight fair when disputes do arise, family members can often preserve their relationships with each other, even if they cannot completely agree on a particular issue. Even when disputes cannot be reconciled, politeness and respect can help to preserve family relationships.

■ FAMILIES, RACIALLY MIXED

Families in which members are of different races are considered racially mixed. In an **interracial marriage**, the husband and wife are of different races. Children born to interracial couples are **biracial**, meaning a mixture of more than one race. In 2000 the census showed that more than one in six adopted children in the United States are a different race from their parents. William Frey, a census analyst from the Brookings Institution in Washington, says that about one in 15 marriages in the United States is interracial. That percentage, according to Frey, is up from one in 23 in 1990 and is approximately 5 percent in 2008.

Most scholars today regard race as a meaningless concept in science because human beings, regardless of their race, are more alike than different. Race, however, has social importance. Because it is a social concept, its meaning varies with the time and the place. For example, the 1870 census divided the population into five races: white, colored (blacks), colored (mulattoes or mixed race), Chinese, and Native American. By 1950, the census categories reflected a different social understanding: white, black, and other.

In 1980, the U.S. census categories reflected the arrival of new groups as a result of a change in the nation's immigration laws. The census now labeled race categories as white, black, Hispanic, Japanese, Chinese, Filipino, Korean, Vietnamese, American Indian, Asian Indian, Hawaiian, Guamanian, Samoan, Eskimo, Aleut, and other. In England that same year, the categories were white, West Indian, African, Arab, Turkish, Chinese, Indian, Pakistani, Bangladeshi, Sri Lankan, and other. In South Africa in 1980, there were only four racial categories: white, African, "coloured" (mixed race) and Asian. Each of these systems of racial classification reflected a different social, economic, and political reality. As social situations change, so do racial categories and other understandings of a racially mixed family.

According to the 2008 census, 6.5 million persons in the United States identified themselves as belonging to more than one race. This number represented slightly more than 2 percent of the population. The 2000 census was the first census to allow individuals to identify themselves as belonging to more than one race. Researcher Donna Nakazawa estimates that by the year 2030, as many as 10 percent of the United States population will consider themselves multiracial.

ACCEPTANCE BY SOCIETY

Although the number of racially mixed families is on the rise, interracial marriage continues to be a source of conflict among some family members and friends. Researcher Peggy Gillespie believes that the debate over adding multiracial categories to the U.S. census forms in 2000 illustrated the deeply embedded role race plays in American life and the way it continues to divide the nation.

Transracial adoption, the adoption of a child of one race by parents of another, has also generated controversy, debate, and discussion. As recently as 1987, 35 states had laws prohibiting the adoption of African-American children by white families. In 1996, President Bill Clinton signed into law a bill that made it illegal to prohibit adoptions based on race.

TEENS SPEAK

I Didn't Even Notice I Was Different

When I was younger, I didn't even notice that I was a different race than the other kids in school. But when I hit fifth grade everyone started to make jokes about my being adopted. At first it didn't really bother me because my parents had always told me how I came to live in my family. After a while the teasing stopped, probably because I tried not to show them that it bothered me. But it did make me more aware of how I am different and how I am the same as everyone else. My parents have always taught me about the country I was born in. I am actually pretty lucky to know so much about life there and life here. I wouldn't change my story; I think I am more open-minded about other people. And I know I don't judge people as much as others judge me. It really helps to have parents that love and accept you for who you are and not how you look.

Both transracial adoptions and interracial marriages are helping to break down racial barriers. Adam Pertman, an adoption expert, attributes an increase in biracial births to the 1967 Supreme Court decision in the case of *Loving v. Virginia*. The decision declared state laws banning interracial marriage unconstitutional. Experts on racially mixed families also suggest that increased interaction among the races at schools and in the workplace further contribute to a greater acceptance of these kinds of families.

Francis Wardle is executive director of the Center for the Study of Biracial Children and adjunct professor at the University of Phoenix-Colorado. He believes that multicultural education in workplaces and schools, teacher training related to issues of diversity, and the promotion of antibias programs nationwide have also led to greater acceptance of racially mixed families.

WHERE DO WE FIT?

Although researchers have documented greater acceptance of racially mixed families, some children still grapple with issues of identity. According to the Center for the Study of Biracial Children, many children are uncertain as to which race they belong. As children mature, they become curious about their racial background, particularly if they must contend with prejudice about their own appearance or the appearance of their parents and siblings. By the time they reach adolescence, children want to know where and how they fit into various social groups and communities. In a study that examined issues in racially mixed families, Elias Cheboud and Chris Downing, researchers from the Capital Region Race Relations Association, found that many children begin to feel societal pressure to choose the identity of one race over another during adolescence.

Even adults may feel that they do not fit in, according to Cheboud and Downing. While few multiracial families feel totally secure, fitting in is becoming easier, experts say. Biracial activist Matt Kelley insists that most families can fit in without choosing sides.

Q & A

Question: How do most biracial children identify themselves?

Answer: As a result of a trend toward increased tolerance nationwide, children are more open about their multiracial background, according to Francis Wardle, executive director of the Center for the Study of Biracial Children. While identity issues may continue for some biracial children, more and more children feel comfortable identifying themselves as racially mixed or talking freely of their experience growing up in a racially mixed family.

IMPACT ON TEENS

While some teens struggle with issues of identity relating to their multiracial background, many do not. In fact, some teens say that the expectation that they will have difficulty is problematic in and of itself. Teens who seek support at the Center for the Study of Biracial Children say that it is frustrating when people expect them to have problems just because of race. Most often the issues they struggle with have more to do with being a teenager than with anything else.

But other teens are uncomfortable with the way their peers react to their biracial identity. They point to feelings of rejection from their peer group, not being taken seriously by others, being subjected to intolerant remarks, and exclusion from social events as particularly troublesome.

The identity issues and the feelings of exclusion that some biracial children describe can lead to behavioral problems, according to the Oregon Alliance of Children's Programs that is part of the juvenile justice system. The group conducted a survey in 2002 that shows that the fastest-growing segment of youths entering the criminal justice system are multiracial youths. The survey also found that many of the children that enter the system have been victimized in some way. Kelly, founder of the Maven Foundation, a non-profit organization aimed at raising awareness about multiracial children and their concerns, says more resources need to be created that celebrate multiracial youths and inform parents and educators about their issues.

With numbers of biracial teens on the rise, many teens date people of other races. Some of these teens cannot understand why their parents who are accepting of racially mixed friendships draw the line at interracial dating. This phenomenon, experts say, illustrates how much further society needs to go to accept racially mixed relationships of all kinds.

See also: Adoption; Family, The New

FURTHER READING

Childs, Erica. *Fade to Black and White: Interracial Images in Popular Culture.* Perspectives on a Multiracial America. Lanham, Md.: Rowman and Littlefield, 2009.

Davis, Bonnie. *The Biracial and Multiracial Student Experience: A Journey to Racial Literacy*. Thousand Oaks, Calif.: Corwin, A SAGE Publishing Company, 2009.

Felder, David. *Raising Biracial Children: Role-Play Peacegame*. Tallahassee, Fla.: Wellington Press, 2010.

Simon, Rita. *In Their Siblings' Voices: White Non-Adopted Siblings Talk About Their Experiences Being Raised with Black and Biracial Brothers and Sisters*. New York: Columbia University Press, 2009.

Smith, Earl. *Interracial Relationships in the 21st Century*. Durham, N.C.: Carolina Academic Press, 2009.

■ FAMILY, THE NEW

The traditional family in the United States has long been a nuclear family—two parents and their unmarried children. Today, fewer children live in such families. More and more children grow up in extended families, single-parent families, blended families, alternative families, or culturally or racially mixed families. An extended family consists of three or more generations. Alternative families may include parents who are gay or lesbian, bisexual, or transgender. In a culturally or racially mixed family, family members may differ from one another in language, ethnicity, religion, or race.

EXTENDED FAMILIES

An extended family consists of three or more generations who share a household. One example of an extended family is one in which a widowed grandmother lives with her married daughter, son-in-law, and grandchildren. The grandmother may help to raise the children while the parents are working. Extended families may live together for a variety of reasons—to save money, help raise children, or care for a member who is ill. Sometimes grandparents take care of their grandchildren full time if the children's parents cannot.

The 2000 U.S. census showed that 2.3 million households had an adult living with a parent. This arrangement is most common among immigrants and in cities with housing shortages and high costs. *America's Families and Living Arrangements: 2008* is a collection of 2008 statistics from the Current Population Survey (CPS) on family and nonfamily households, characteristics of single-parent families, living arrangements of children, and data on married and unmarried couples. The CPS has been conducted annually since 1940. Findings from the 2008 CPS show that about 9 percent of all children (6.6 million) lived in a household that included a grandparent. Twenty-three percent of children living with a grandparent had no parent present. When assessing racial differences, the CPS data show 6 percent of white non-Hispanic children lived in a household with a grandparent present, compared with 10 percent of Hispanic children, and 14 percent of both Asian and black children.

In the United States, according to social worker George W. Doherty in his report *Extended Families,* immigrant families are often extended by choice and necessity. His research shows, for example, that many Mexican-American parents rely on the support of their extended family. Family members share not only child care, but also the care of elderly relatives.

TEENS SPEAK

It's Different Growing Up in an Extended Family

I'm Chinese American, and I can tell you that leaving home at a certain age is not a part of Chinese culture. The Chinese believe that a child's leaving home is based on his or her maturity. My parents believe that it is better to not leave home until you marry! Otherwise you are not being respectful. Your parents would think you don't love them. Even when you graduate from college, your parents still must take care of you. So I can't move out until I marry, even though I've told my parents that they will save money if I leave. I have told them many times that I will always love them—even if I leave home.

In a statement in 2003, President George W. Bush praised families who choose to take care of elderly or ill relatives at home:

Millions of Americans make extraordinary efforts every day to care for loved ones who are elderly, chronically ill, or disabled. These caregivers make many sacrifices to improve the lives of their loved ones. Through their love, dedication, and courage, these compassionate children, parents, spouses, grandparents, and extended family members strengthen and preserve the importance of family and reflect the true character of our nation.

Living in an extended family can be difficult because individuals have less privacy and less independence than in a nuclear family. It may also be hard to provide everyone with the attention he or she requires. According to a 2001 guide to extended family relationships published by *Resources for Living,* a counseling group that works with many such families, these tensions can be reduced by setting clear boundaries.

ALTERNATIVE FAMILIES

Alternative families are those created by unmarried heterosexual couples, homosexual couples, bisexuals, or transgender persons. Children in such families may be a result of artificial insemination or adoption.

Q & A

Question: Are gay people allowed to adopt?

Answer: Many state laws allow any adult person to adopt. However, even in those states, courts may not be willing to allow gays to adopt. Florida does not permit gays or lesbians to adopt, and Mississippi and Utah allow gay singles to adopt but not gay couples.

According to the U.S. Census Bureau, in 1998 about 167,000 gay parents were rearing children under 15 years of age. Results from the 2008 American Community Survey indicate that at least 400,000–500,000 gay or lesbian parents live with children in the United States.

Because the state does not always recognize relationships in alternative families, these families often have to draw up legal documents that protect the rights of family members to inherit property, participate in medical decision making, and share in the guardianship of children.

For example, prior to starting a family, lawyer Elizabeth Schwartz suggests that prospective gay parents make a formal agreement in which they spell out their intent to cooperate with each other in rearing a child. Schwartz also advises these parents to formally state what their respective monetary contributions will be and what should happen if one partner dies or the couple decides to separate.

Parents in alternative relationships often experience discrimination by the larger society and even their own families. Many turn to parenting groups and other support systems to help them make up for that loss.

Fact Or Fiction?

It is safer for children who are part of an alternative family to remain silent about their parents.

The Facts: According to the Family Pride Coalition's *Issues and News* 2004, children in alternative families do need to be careful before they speak openly about their living arrangements. Doing so in some situations may be dangerous. However, not talking about their families may imply that something is wrong with the way they live. It is crucial for schools to foster safe places for children to talk about their families and to know that their families are okay.

According to a review of research in the 1990s by Geri R. Donenberg, a professor of psychiatry at the University of Illinois at Chicago, children reared in alternative families, such as those headed by gays and lesbians, are very similar to those who grow up with heterosexual parents. For example, the American Academy of Pediatrics studied children of gay parents in 2002 in terms of the psychosocial aspects of family health. The group found no significant differences between children of gay parents compared to children of heterosexual parents. A review of recent studies assessing the effect of gay parenting on children, published in the *Journal of Marriage and Family,* determined that little effect was found between the social and psychological success of children and parent gender.

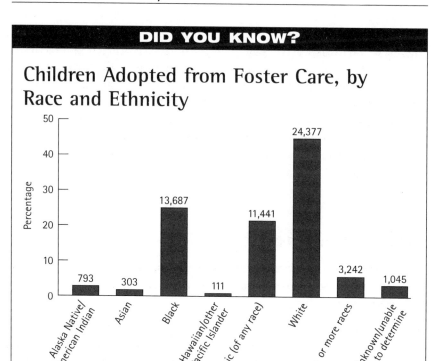

DID YOU KNOW?

Children Adopted from Foster Care, by Race and Ethnicity

The racial makeup of the modern American family is increasingly diverse. Adoption is one way in which the diversity of family members grows. As of 2008, although the largest percentage of children who were adopted from the public foster care system were white, 25 percent were black, followed by 21 percent Hispanic, followed by Alaskan or American Indian children, followed by Asian children, and then by Hawaiian or other Pacific Islanders.

Source: Adoption and Foster Care Analysis and Reporting System (AFCARS), U.S. Department of Health and Human Services, Administration for Children and Families, Administration on Children, Youth and Families, Children's Bureau, October 2007-September 2008.

CULTURALLY AND RACIALLY MIXED FAMILIES

In a mixed family, family members differ in race, culture, and/or religion. Interracial and multicultural families have much to share but may also have to overcome many challenges in order to understand each other.

According to the 2008 Census—the first to allow Americans to define themselves as multiracial or multicultural—6.5 million people described themselves as multiracial, about 2.2 percent of the population. Current projections by the Census Bureau suggest that by 2050, people of European descent will constitute about 53 percent of the population, while Hispanics, African Americans, and Asians will make up 25, 14, and 8 percent, respectively.

Some multiracial and multicultural families experience discrimination and intolerance. As diversity has increased in the United States, so has acceptance of these families.

To summarize, not all families have the same living arrangements. Families in the United States today include extended families and alternative families as well as culturally or racially mixed families.

See also: Families, Racially Mixed; Gay Parents; Religion and the Family

FURTHER READING

Boenke, Mary. *Trans Forming Families.* 3rd ed. Washington, D.C.: PFLAG Transgender Network, 2009.

Epstein, Rachel. *Who's Your Daddy?: And Other Writings on Queer Parenting.* Ontario, Canada: Sumach Press, 2009.

Fields, Julianna. *Gay and Lesbian Parents.* The Changing Face of Modern Families. Broomall, Pa.: Mason Crest Publishers, 2009.

■ FAMILY, THE TRADITIONAL

A traditional family consists of a married couple and their unmarried children; it is sometimes also called a nuclear family. Parents generally play traditional gender roles, with the man assuming responsibility for financially supporting the family and the woman for maintaining the household and caring for the children.

Many factors—including a high divorce rate, changing economic conditions, and the increased participation of women in the labor force—have combined to make the traditional family only one of many family structures in the United States today. As family forms become more diverse, the traditional family is becoming less common.

DO THEY STILL WORK?

The average life cycle of the traditional family can be inferred from census and other data. When the couple marries, the man is 26 and the woman is 24. Two years later, the woman gives birth to the first of the couple's two children. The second child is born two years later. For the next 20 years, the husband works outside the home, while the wife cares for their home and children. When the youngest child leaves home, the wife is 48 and the husband is 50. They become "empty nesters." The man continues to work until he is 65. He is about 74 years old when he dies. The woman will probably live five years longer than he did, dying at 79.

In the 1950s, about two-thirds of American children grew up in families that fit this portrait of a mother, father, and their children. In a traditional family, gender roles for husband and wife were clearly defined. The husband provided the income; the wife stayed home and cared for the family. The children spent their days in school. Not only was the husband the breadwinner, but he was also responsible for tasks defined as "man's work." "Man's work" usually included handling the family finances, making home and car repairs, and acting as the chief disciplinarian for the children. The wife was expected to perform "women's work," which usually included cleaning the house, cooking, sewing and mending, and child care. Children were expected to attend school and to spend their free time in play.

By 2000, this picture had changed. The percentage of married-couple households dropped from 78 percent of all households in 1950 to just 52 percent in 2000. According to census data, more people are opting to live alone and many others are delaying marriage and childbirth. The percentage of households occupied by one person increased from 11 percent in 1950 to almost 26 percent in 2000. Family size also decreased in the late 1900s. Between 1970 and 2000, the number of households with five or more people dropped from 21 percent to 10 percent. The percentage of married couples with children also declined. In 1960, about 60 percent of married couples had at least one child; by 1990, less than half had a child.

Data from the National Center for Health Statistics (NCHS) also show that the divorce rate increased between 1950 and 1980, leveling off in the 1990s. By 2009, almost half of all marriages ended in divorce, with 20 percent of marriages ending within three years. The high divorce rate means that more than 60 percent of children live in a single-parent household before they are 18. Blended and reblended families are becoming more common as divorced parents remarry—half of them more than once. Census Bureau data also indicates that **cohabitation**, the practice of living together without marriage, is becoming more common. In 2009, 6.6 million unmarried couples were cohabitating, many (1.8 million) with their biological children. According to 2008 Census Bureau data for unmarried couples, 5.6 million couples were heterosexual and just under 600,000 were homosexual. Within same-sex couples, more than 500,000 were males and 270,600 were females. Overall, in 2008, greater than 55 million opposite-sex couples were married.

Other data from the NCHS show wide fluctuations in the **fertility rate**—the average number of children a woman has in her lifetime. In the late 1950s, the average woman gave birth to 3.5 children. The fertility rate dropped to a low of 1.8 births per woman in 1972, then climbed slightly and stayed at between 2.0 and 2.1 births from the early 1990s through 2003. The NCHS data from 2007 show the number of births was 4.3 million, which represents a birthrate of 14.3 per 1,000 births. During the same period, the fertility rate for women ages 15 to 44 was 69.5 per 1,000 women. The percentage of unmarried women who gave birth to children climbed from 5 percent in 1960 to 39.7 percent in 2007.

Gender roles are also becoming more fluid as more and more married women enter the workforce. According to a report issued in November 1999 by the National Opinion Research Center at the University of Chicago, attitudes toward married women's participation in the workforce changed dramatically in the last quarter of the 20th century. In 1972, 67 percent approved of a wife working even if her husband could support her. By the 1990s, that percentage rose to 83 percent. In 2008, according to the Bureau of Labor Statistics, both husband and wife worked outside the home in 51.4 percent of married-couple families. Married women today are more likely to pursue careers as part of their life goals, while men are spending more time with their children and performing household tasks. The percentage of households in which women work outside the home and men are the primary caretakers of children rose from 2 percent in 1972 to almost 6.9 percent in 2008.

Sociologists and demographers attribute many of these shifts to changes in norms, values, laws, the economy, and the health of the elderly. As divorce, single parenthood, and remarriage become more common, the traditional family becomes only one of many possible family types. In November 2000 sociologist Jay D. Teachman and his colleagues at Western Washington University published the results of a study that examined the effects of economic patterns on marriage and family stability. The study, which appeared in the *Journal of Marriage and the Family,* suggests that a woman's income is becoming more important as a source of economic stability. Teachman's research builds on earlier work by other researchers, including sociologists and demographers. These researchers maintain that as women achieve greater economic independence, they are less likely to stay in unhappy marriages. Another factor is cited by sociologist Valerie Oppenheimer. She points out that men's earning power has declined, leaving fewer families able to survive on the income of a single wage earner.

DO THEY STILL EXIST?

The traditional family may be a rapidly disappearing entity. According to data from the 2000 census, fewer people are living in nuclear families today than ever before. In 1970, married couples who lived with their own children made up 40 percent of households in the United States. By 2009, that number had dropped to 25 percent. This figure includes blended families, so the percentage of families that include a father, mother, and their mutual offspring is probably even lower.

TEENS SPEAK

I Thought Families Didn't Come Any More Traditional Than Mine

My family is what the experts would call a "traditional family." My parents just celebrated their 25th anniversary. They married when they were both in their early 20s. For as long as I can remember, my father has worked—he's an emergency room physician at the local hospital—and my mother has taken care of our house, my brother, my sister, and me. She cleans the house and drives us to soccer practice, piano and ballet lessons, and everywhere else we go.

To someone looking in from the outside, families don't come any more traditional than mine. In comparison to my friends' families, we're almost "embarrassingly normal." About half of my friends' parents have divorced at least once. Some of my friends live with just one parent, stepparents, step-stepparents, or grandparents. My friend Michelle has two mothers.

But anyone living in my family would quickly see that we are rather nontraditional. Not only does my mother clean the house, she also does most of the home and car maintenance. She changes the oil on both her car and dad's, fixes leaky faucets and other problems around the house, mows the lawn, and takes out the garbage every week. She's also an environmental activist. I started going to peace rallies when I was still in my stroller. Dad couldn't fix a leaky faucet if you offered him a million dollars, but he loves to cook. He does most of the cooking whenever he's not working a 24-hour shift at the hospital. He also loves, believe it or not, to sew. He made most of our clothes when we were younger, and he still sews curtains and other things for the house as well as the tents we use each summer for our family vacation.

According to Stephanie Coontz, professor of history and family studies at Evergreen State College in Olympia, Washington, the question might not be whether the traditional family still exists but whether it ever existed at all. In *The Way We Never Were: American Families and the Nostalgia Trap,* Coontz argues that the portrait of the 1950s traditional family was true for very few people. Coontz points out that during the 1950s, divorce rates were low, but more than 2 million people lived separately while remaining legally married. Married women were more likely to suffer depression and anxiety than working mothers. Many states did not allow married women to sign contracts, secure credit cards or loans, or serve on juries.

Unmarried mothers were forced to marry or they were shipped off to another town to give birth and then give their babies up for adoption. The number of pregnant brides doubled in the 1950s, while the number of infants born to unmarried mothers and available for adoption rose 80 percent between 1944 and 1955. Coontz suggests that the post–World War II economic boom led to a strong labor market and relatively high wages for men. In this economic environment, many men could support a family and buy a home without help from other family members. Still, 25 percent of the population lived below the poverty line, and one-third of white American families could not subsist on the income of only one working adult. Children were more likely to go hungry, and people over 65 were more likely to be poor than they were in 2008. Coontz also points out that the discrepancy between the myth of the American nuclear family and the reality of family life was even more apparent for people of various ethnic backgrounds. More than half of all African-American families lived in poverty, even when both parents worked.

Fact Or Fiction?

"Latchkey children" suffer greatly.

The Facts: About 5 million children between the ages of five and 13 are home on a regular basis without direct adult supervision. Most of these children are the sons and daughters of white, middle-class parents who live in suburban or rural areas. These "latchkey children"—the name comes from the fact that they often carry a house key so they can let themselves into their homes—may experience both positive and negative effects. Latchkey children may be more independent and self-reliant, have less stereotypical gender-role expectations of mothers, interact more with friends, help out more with household duties, and be better able to care for themselves than children who always have an adult in the house. However, they also may be fearful and apprehensive at being left alone, especially if they are left alone in an environment in which crime is high.

For most of the last 2,000 years, mothers have spent almost as much time in paid employment as they have raising children. Coontz argues that the idea that women's main function was to mother was a relatively recent one. Not until the 19th century did white, middle-class women withdraw from the workforce, prompted partly by a cultural ideal that equated womanhood with motherhood and a woman's leisure time with her husband's success. Women in low-income families have always worked outside the home, usually for lower wages than men. Children also contributed significantly to family incomes. Coontz suggests that after child labor laws were imposed in the 1960s, married women immediately began to reenter the workforce. By 1997, only 15 percent of families were supported solely by a male.

SINGLE-BREADWINNER FAMILIES

Families in which only one spouse works are becoming the exception, not the rule. Census Bureau data shows that in 1960, 42 percent of all families were supported solely by a male. By 2009, the male was the sole breadwinner in only 20 percent of families.

The financial adjustments

Most families that depend on a single earner have a limited income. If one spouse has been working and decides to leave the labor force to care for the couple's children, the family faces a drop in income at the same time that it encounters the increased expense of a child in the household. While families in which the working partner earns high wages may not experience a dramatic drop in income, most families in the middle-income range may have more difficulty adjusting to a lower income level. For families in lower-income brackets, it may not be financially possible for one spouse to stay at home.

Single-income living usually requires careful budgeting and planning, starting with the calculation of the lost income. According to experts, those considering whether to become a single-income family should calculate the net income that will be lost when one spouse leaves work after subtracting taxes, the costs of child care, commuting, work clothes, meals out, and extras like office parties and gifts. The reduction in income may affect all family members.

Income-earning spouses in single-earner families may feel that the income that they contribute to the family belongs to them. When both partners work and contribute financially to a family, money is often shared equally. But when only one spouse is contributing financially, that spouse may feel entitled to make financial decisions without consulting his or her partner. Conversely, the person who is not working outside the home may feel he or she needs to ask permission to spend money, even on necessities. The change in the couple's financial relationship may be a source of stress to both partners.

The couple's choice may be affected by the number of children in the household. The more children a couple has, the greater the child care demands and the more expensive it is to provide child care. In a 1996 study published in the *Journal of Marriage and the Family,* sociologist Stacy J. Rogers examined the effect of mothers' work hours on marital quality. She found that full-time employment of mothers in large families was associated with less marital happiness and more conflict.

In 2004 Rogers published another study of family economics— "Dollars, Dependency, and Divorce: Four Perspectives on the Role of Wives' Income"—in *Journal of Marriage and the Family.* After interviewing 2,033 couples in 1980 and again in 1983, 1988, 1992, and 1997, Rogers found that the greater the difference between spouse's incomes, the greater the chance that couple would divorce. Conversely, couples that were happy and equally rewarded by their work were less likely to divorce. Rogers concluded that when women are employed, the increased family income can enhance marital stability and contribute to the family's economic security.

Cultural pressures

In a society that equates individual identity with work, being a stay-at-home parent can be challenging for both men and women. According to the National Association of At-home Mothers, parents who choose to stay home and devote their energies to raising children and maintaining a home may be pressured from friends and family to work outside the home. They may also face questions about their decision to become "full-time parents."

Women who choose to focus their energies on their family and home may be stigmatized, in an odd reversal of cultural stereotypes of the 1950s. In the 1950s, the married mother who chose to work was often considered selfish and inattentive to her children. In 1947, a best-selling book, *The Modern Woman,* claimed that the idea of the independent woman was a "contradiction in terms," and warned that women who wanted equal economic and educational opportunities were engaged in a "ritualistic castration" of men. While most of this myth has been dispelled, women who choose employment may still experience criticism for spending less time with their children. But the married mother who chooses not to work may also find herself apologizing for being "just" a mom.

Men who choose to stay at home may find the adjustment even more difficult, mostly because men have been reared to identify themselves as providers for their families. Since the 1960s, researchers have been examining the ways that married women's participation in the labor force affects families. Many of these studies, including a 2001 study of the effects of wives' income on marital stability and happiness by sociologists Stacy J. Rogers and Danielle D. DeBoer, indicate that the ability to financially support a family continues to be an important aspect of men's well-being. Rogers and DeBoer's study, "Changes in Wives' Income: Effects on Marital Happiness, Psychological Well-being, and the Risk of Divorce," was published in the *Journal of Marriage and the Family*. The researchers found that when women's incomes rose, their marital happiness and well-being increased. However, when women contributed a greater percentage of the total household income—40 to 50 percent—men's well-being decreased, even when the men did not subscribe to traditional gender roles. Rogers and DeBoer concluded that the decrease in men's well-being reflected continued emphasis on men as the family breadwinner, despite increasing support for nontraditional gender roles by both women and men.

WHO STAYS HOME?

Traditionally, the man has been the primary economic provider in the family, while women assumed responsibility for child care and household tasks. While this division of labor is still prevalent in traditional families, other families in the United States today opt for different arrangements—including one in which the woman works and the man stays home. As gender roles become less defined by gender, so does the division of labor within households. The Census Bureau reports that in 2009, 158,000 fathers stayed at home to care for their children under the age of 15. These fathers chose not to work primarily so they could care for the children while their wives worked outside the home.

For the most part, however, it is women who stay home to care for the children. The gender wage gap may affect the family's decision about who stays home. Estimates from the Institute for Women's Policy (IWPR) research show that women earn only 71 cents for every dollar that men earn, often even when they are employed in similar jobs. IWPR's analysis of census data showed that even during the peak earning years of ages 45–54, women earned 68 percent of what men earned in 1998.

That discrepancy persists even after factors such as education and work experience are taken into account. Data compiled by the American Federation of Labor and Congress of Industrial Organizations (AFL-CIO) show that in 2003, women in professional and technical occupations earned almost 27 percent less than men, while women in sales occupations earned 38 percent less. One of the largest differences was among physicians. Female physicians and surgeons earned 41 percent less than their male counterparts. According to a

2004 study from IWPR, *Still a Man's Labor Market: The Long-Term Earnings Gap,* on average a woman who was in her prime earning years between 1983 and 1998 earned $273,592 during that 15-year period; the average man earned $722,693. IWPR researchers say the male-female wage gap appears to have three underlying causes. First, women are more likely to work in lower-paying jobs such as nursing and teaching. Second, women may not work as many hours per week as men. Third, women are less likely to advocate for increases in their own pay. According to the IWPR in 2009, the median weekly earnings of female full-time workers were $657, compared with male median weekly earnings of $819. Based on these data, the ratio of women's to men's median weekly earnings was 80.2, slightly higher than in 2008 but still below the historical high of 81.0 in 2005.

In every single-income family, the decision of who will stay home is a very personal one. The woman may be a more skilled worker or more highly educated than the man, she may have a job that pays more and has better benefits, or she may want to work because she finds that work contributes to her own well-being and ability to mother. The man may identify strongly with the traditional male role of provider and be unwilling or ill-suited to being the primary child-care provider.

SHARING RESPONSIBILITIES

For many couples, the home is becoming a place of shared responsibility and caring, rather than the site of "women's work." In a 1987 study of 640 white, middle-class parents, psychologist Rosalind Barnett and sociologist Grace Baruch examined factors that affected fathers' participation in child care. They found that a father's participation in child-care tasks was linked to a number of variables. The more hours the mother worked per week, the more likely he was to assist with child care. A mother who expected help from her husband got more help than those who did not expect and ask for the help. Fathers who were unhappy with the fathering they had received as children tended to be more involved in caring for their own children. Those fathers also spent more time with their children when they were small and devoted more time to their sons than to their daughters. As the number of children in the family increased, so did the percentage of time that fathers interacted with their children. Finally, fathers who were employed but worked fewer hours spent more time caring for their children. However, unemployment made it less likely that fathers would spend time with their children.

Although the difference between the amount of time women and men spend performing housework and child care is decreasing, women still do more family work than men. Several studies, including a 2001 study of the relationship between domestic labor and marital satisfaction published in the *Journal of Marriage and the Family*, show that both employed and unemployed women in all income brackets spend significantly more time doing housework and caring for children than men do. Sociologist Daphne Stevens and her colleagues at Utah State University found that whether they work outside the home or not, women tend to have more responsibility for children. Women are more likely to plan and carry out decisions regarding children's care and to spend more time caring for their children. Yet the researchers found that the happiest couples didn't necessarily divide household tasks equally. The happiest couples in their study had developed a mutually agreed-upon division of household labor and financial responsibilities. That agreement, not the 50/50 division of household labor, had the most influence on marital happiness. The "adult worker family" has replaced the male breadwinner/housewife family over the past generation as reported by a 2009 study in the journal *Community Work & Family*. This model defines shared responsibilities within the household by both male and female. Responsibilities include household work, child care, and providing economic resources.

Men and women are more likely to share home responsibilities when they are somewhat egalitarian in their beliefs about gender roles in relationships. Yet segregation of home responsibilities seems to persist even in egalitarian relationships.

Q & A

Question: Can a woman be a feminist and still be in a traditional family?

Answer: Feminists do not object to women's traditional roles within families but believe that women should be able to choose whether or not to play those roles. Many feminists argue that the work that women have traditionally done should be valued as much as the work that men traditionally do. For instance, if a husband wants to stay home and take care of his children instead of pursuing a career, that choice should be recognized as valid and valuable. Likewise, when women choose to stay home and provide care to their children, their activities should be recognized as equal in importance to her husband's work outside the home.

This segregation of tasks may stem partly from gender-role stereotypes, which deeply affect both men and women. Men or women who consciously or unconsciously hold traditional gender-role beliefs may inhibit one another from sharing household tasks. Even men who want to spend more time with their children may find that their wives are reluctant to give up the control. The mother may see family work as her domain. Some women act as "gatekeepers," preventing men from more involvement with children and household tasks. After studying this phenomenon, sociologists Sarah Allen and Alan Hawkins defined maternal gatekeeping as "a collection of beliefs and behaviors that ultimately inhibit a collaborative effort between men and women in family work by limiting men's opportunities for learning and growing through caring for home and children." In a 1999 study of 1,500 women published in the *Journal of Marriage and the Family,* Allen and Hawkins found that 25 percent engaged in some kind of gatekeeping behaviors. Such gatekeeping activities, they argue, provide barriers to fathers' involvement in housework and child care.

Once the most common family structure, the traditional family—consisting of a mother, father, and their biological children, in which the father is the breadwinner and the mother cares for the home and children—has become increasingly less common in the United States. The decrease in the percentage of traditional families stems from many factors, including increasing rates of divorce, single parenthood, and remarriage; women's increased participation in the labor force; and changing gender role expectations. Families in which only one spouse works are becoming the exception rather than the rule. As more married women work outside the home, taking on some of the financial responsibilities for the family, many couples are dividing household tasks more equally.

See also: Day Care; Divorce and Families; Families, Blended; Families, Racially Mixed; Family, The New; Family Traditions; Marriage and Family, Changes in; Single-Parent Families

FURTHER READING
Gersen, Kathleen. *The Unfinished Revolution: How a New Generation Is Reshaping Family, Work, and Gender in America.* New York: Oxford University Press, 2009.

■ FAMILY BOUNDARIES

Within a family, something indicating a border or limit. Family boundaries come in a variety of forms. They can be something physical, such as a bedroom door, or intangible, such as the time of your curfew. The door represents a boundary between a public space and a private space. Your curfew represents a limit in time after which you must be home. Family boundaries are important for healthy communication, nurturing relationships, and privacy.

BOUNDARIES BETWEEN PARENTS AND CHILDREN

Each member of your family has an important role to play. Whether you live with your mom and dad, a single parent, stepparent, foster parents, or other legal guardian, their first responsibility is your well-being. You ought to be their first priority. It is their job to make sure you're eating all the right foods (including your vegetables), receiving a good education, getting enough exercise, and making sure your friends are a positive influence in your life, not a negative one. Your parent is there to guide you in the right direction, discipline you when you have stepped out of line, and comfort you when you're sad.

Some parents may choose to involve their children in important decisions. This can be a good thing and is often a sign that they recognize a certain level of maturity in you. However, it is important to remember that your parents are not supposed to treat you like their best friend, confiding in you about every worry.

Sadly, parental boundaries frequently are overstepped, sometimes resulting in emotional, physical, and sexual abuse. According to data collected by the U.S. Department of Health and Human Services on child abuse victims, 79.9 percent of perpetrators were the parents of the victims.

PRIVACY

Everyone needs alone time. This is especially true for adults. The door to your parents' bedroom is a boundary with special rules. When the door is open, it is important to announce yourself before entering. If the door is closed, always knock and wait for a reply. Never enter without an invitation. In the end, if you cross this boundary without invitation, it will most likely be you who is embarrassed!

As a growing teen, you are increasingly aware of your own need for privacy. Unlike when you were a little kid, you do not want to share everything with your parents and that's okay. However, it is important to realize that your parents may have different ideas about how much privacy you need. Again, a parent's number one priority is your safety and well-being. For example, your mom has the right to monitor your computer use because you are a minor. If she feels you might be in danger, it is her responsibility to check it out. In order to avoid any sticky situations, talk to your parents about what is appropriate and what is not.

Fact Or Fiction?

Siblings of the opposite sex legally must have separate bedrooms by the age of puberty.

The Facts: There is no legislation in any state that requires siblings of the opposite sex to maintain separate bedrooms. Families with multiple children do not always have the financial means to afford a residence with separate bedrooms for each child. With that said, it is customary and advisable for adolescent siblings of the opposite sex to have separate bedrooms.

The only instance in which this is legally enforceable is in foster homes. According to the Division of Child and Family Services in the state of Illinois, in a foster home, "Children under six years of age may share a bedroom with related children of the opposite sex who are also under age six if each child is provided with a separate bed or crib," and "Unrelated children under two years of age may share a bedroom with children of the opposite sex who are also under the age of two if each child is provided a separate bed or crib." In other words, adolescent children of the opposite sex, whether they are related or not, may not share a bedroom in a foster care situation.

Part of gaining more privacy is that it must be earned. The best way to build a trusting relationship with your parents is to talk to them. Tell them who your friends are and what you like to do on the weekends. By maintaining an open relationship with parents, they will be more likely to trust you and respect your privacy. If you constantly come home late or get into trouble at school, your parents will question your level of maturity and thus your ability to make good decisions in difficult situations.

Boundaries you should expect as a teen:

- Your parents have the right to know your whereabouts.
- As a legal minor, you are subject to the rules of your parents. This means obeying the time they give for your curfew.
- The older we get, the more privacy we need. It is good to set aside time during the day in which you can be alone listening to music, reading, writing, or even daydreaming. A journal or diary is a good way to jot down your private thoughts.

BOUNDARIES OUTSIDE OF THE HOME

Every family is a little different. Maybe for you, the word family simply refers to your siblings and parents and grandparents. Perhaps for the person sitting next to you in homeroom family includes old friends of his parents in his "family." However one defines family, it seems that there is a special kind of line that people draw between those who are in and those who are outside of our family. Your family ought to be a place you can turn when you have questions or concerns about the world outside your doors.

It is perfectly healthy to have a trusted adult outside of the home to whom you can turn when you have questions you think your parents cannot answer or questions you might not feel comfortable asking your parents. According to the Search Institute, having several relationships with supportive adults outside the home is one of 40 Developmental Assets. These are defined as "concrete, positive, common sense experiences and qualities that provide understanding of what young people need to succeed and be healthy," and they "have the power to protect youth from negative behaviors such as substance abuse, violence, and early sexual activity."

Whatever shape they take, family boundaries can be seen as rules that ought to be followed in order for everyone in your home to live happily and comfortably. Like any rule, there will be consequences if disobeyed. Have you ever heard the term *crossing the line?* This generally refers to an incident in which a person has overstepped appropriate boundaries, resulting in potentially abusive behavior. Understanding what healthy family boundaries are will help you grow into a healthy individual.

See also: Arguments in the Family; Family Rules; Violence in the Family.

FURTHER READING
Buron, Kari Dunn. *A 5 Is Against the Law! Social Boundaries: Straight Up!* Shawnee Mission, Kans.: Autism Asperger Publishing Company, 2007.
Nelson, Margaret K. *Who's Watching?: Daily Practices of Surveillance Among Contemporary Families.* Nashville, Tenn.: Vanderbilt University Press, 2009.
Shea, Kitty. *Teens in the U.S.A.* Mancato, Minn.: Compass Point Books, 2008.

■ FAMILY COUNSELING
A form of therapy that focuses on the interactions between and among family members with the understanding that a family is a system or a team. A family is a whole made up of distinct individuals. The goal of a good counselor is to build bridges of communication between its members while highlighting the family's strengths and weaknesses.

Counseling can involve the parents, children, and extended family. Reasons for seeking family counseling may vary. They may include marital problems, substance abuse by a family member, or even a death in the family. The counselor's main goal is to help the family communicate in order to work through a crisis.

HOW FAMILY COUNSELING WORKS
Many counselors do not see the family all at once. Instead, they work with individual parts—the couple, a child—to remedy specific dysfunctions.

If we think about the family as a team, then it is useful to view the counselor or therapist as a coach. A good coach will understand how the game ought to be played and why things go wrong. Sometimes all the coach needs to do is point out where an adjustment is needed; other times he or she needs to sit down with the team and start from scratch. If a team member does not know how to throw a ball, how can she win a game? It is the same with families: If people never learned how to communicate effectively, how can they expect to be understood or understand the needs of those around them? It is the counselor's job to discuss the problems and needs, realistic and unrealistic; to isolate problem areas; and to help the family and the individuals in it improve their reactions to each other. Improvement may focus on such issues as communication, anger management, money, rivalries, and numerous other issues.

Depending on the counselor, counseling can last anywhere from six sessions to years of therapy. Many counselors assign homework as a tool to further the progress of the family outside of the counseling session. This may include having a family meeting during which parents and children can voice their concerns and then report back to the counselor.

Fact Or Fiction?

Children break up marriages.

The Facts: When families break apart, many children feel as though it is their fault. This is untrue. Rather, it is often the parents' lack of family management that leads to disruption and disorder. Although differences in parenting styles and child rearing practices may lead to spousal conflict, the child is not responsible for a failed marriage. Counseling that involves the whole family is a beneficial way to highlight the different roles and responsibilities of each family member. It is important for children and teens to understand that it is not their job to fix adult problems. Instead, they should focus on doing well in school, being helpful around the house, and most important, just being kids!

TECHNIQUES

One popular approach used by many family counselors is *family systems theory.* Every family, no matter how big or how small, is made up of people of different ages, personalities, and experiences. Each member of the family has an important role to play. When rules are ignored or roles are mixed up, problems arise. This is because the family is a

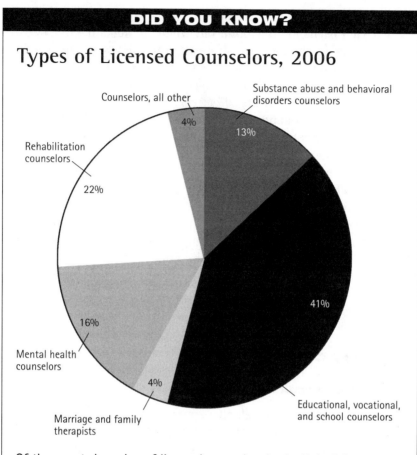

DID YOU KNOW?

Types of Licensed Counselors, 2006

Counselors, all other — 4%

Substance abuse and behavioral disorders counselors — 13%

Rehabilitation counselors — 22%

Educational, vocational, and school counselors — 41%

Mental health counselors — 16%

Marriage and family therapists — 4%

Of the reported number of licensed counselors in the United States, about 4 percent are classified as marriage and family counselors. In other words, of the 636,000 U.S. counselors, 24,701 deal specifically with family counseling.

Source: *Occupational Outlook Handbook*, 2008-09 Edition. U.S. Bureau of Labor Statistics, 2009.

system. Imagine what it would be like if, one day, Jupiter decided to change its course and randomly orbited the Sun. This would probably disrupt the solar system and could cause many problems.

According to the authors of "Core Techniques in Family Therapy," in *Integrating Family Therapy: Handbook of Family Psychology and Systems Theory*, there are several main techniques or interventions that modern family counselors apply during therapy sessions, regardless of which particular major theory they may support.

Sometimes a counselor may look at the way a family is set up and how it changes. While a therapist certainly will take into consideration the initial reason the family has sought counseling, such as a divorce, he or she will not focus on that one issue alone. By looking at the big picture—relationships between members from grandparents to infants, major life events, and patterns of behavior—a counselor is able to work toward permanent change that will benefit the entire family. For example, a family may have decided to seek counseling because their 15-year-old son, "Jimmy," has developed a drug problem.

Working with the whole family or individuals, the family counselor will endeavor to build an intimate relationship with each family member in order to gain a clearer understanding of how this family functions. For example,

- Are they open with each other?
- How do the parents generally handle a crisis? What kinds of boundaries are present?

After gaining some insight into the family, a counselor may be able to determine other areas of dysfunction and how this may relate to the current crisis. In this approach, experts view an individual's problem, such as Jimmy's drug use, as stemming from how the family functions as a whole. The counselor working with Jimmy and Jimmy's family will seek ways to bring about productive and lasting change. If the family and the counselor are active in figuring out the major problem areas and devising a plan to improve the members' interactions, then positive growth can occur in a short period of time.

Another approach is using the family of origin, and its functions and dysfunctions, to solve current problems. The focus here is generational and may deal with grandparents and parents and their impact on the family as it now functions. The therapist must determine these various factors and their impact on current family issues.

See also: Arguments and the Family; Family Rules

FURTHER READING

Ambrose, Marylou, and Veronica Deisler. *Investigating Eating Disorders, Anorexia, Bulimia, and Binge Eating: Real Facts for Real Lives.* Berkeley Heights, N.J.: Enslow Publishers, 2010.

Meisel, Abigail. *Investigating Depression and Bipolar Disorder: Real Facts for Real Lives.* Berkeley Heights, N.J.: Enslow Publishers, 2010.

Winston, Robert. *What Goes on in My Head?* New York: DK Publishing, 2010.

■ FAMILY RULES

Family rules are the guidelines for interaction within a family. Rules, limits, and boundaries are necessary for any group of people to live and work together effectively. Rules guide communication and help individuals know what is expected of them and how to treat one another. In family life, parents are responsible for conveying rules of behavior to their children. When rules are clear and communicated effectively, children learn the skills they need to function effectively at home, in school, and in the community. Knowing what to expect and how to act in various settings helps children feel safe and secure.

WHO IS IN CHARGE?

The word *authority* has many meanings. In relation to family life, parents are the authority. They have the power to influence the actions of their children. As the authority figures in the family, parents are responsible for teaching their children to accept limits and act in acceptable ways. As the authority figures, parents make rules, enforce those rules, and guide behavior. Other authority figures in a family may be grandparents or other adults who provide similar guidance.

Jane B. Brooks, author of *The Process of Parenting,* in its seventh edition, says that children are more likely to follow rules when parents define the rules and clearly communicate those rules to their children. Much research exists describing the ways in which parents set and enforce rules. Researcher Nancy Darling studies the role of rules in family life in a 2008 article titled "Individual Differences in Adolescents' Beliefs About the Legitimacy of Parental Authority and Their Own Obligations to Obey," in the journal *Child Development,* in which she explored several different parenting styles. She highlights three approaches to setting rules and enforcing them. The three are generally known as an authoritarian style, a permissive style, and an authoritative style. Each style is characterized by the way in which parents respond to their children emotionally and how parents try to control their children's behavior.

Authoritarian parents tend to be demanding and directive but not responsive. They clearly state family rules and enforce them. Children are expected to obey or accept the consequences of not following the rules. They have little input into those rules. Parents with an authoritarian style provide their children with strict boundaries with little focus on the expression of feelings related to those rules.

Permissive parents are more responsive than demanding. They place more emphasis on the feelings related to the rules and less on establishing firm boundaries. Parents who are permissive are often willing to negotiate the rules with their children and are likely to place little emphasis on strict enforcement of rules.

Authoritative parents are both demanding and responsive. In families where this style is present, the children know and understand their family's standards of behavior. The children are likely to have some input into rules and family decisions, but adults have the ultimate authority.

The research on parenting style reveals that the way in which rules are established and enforced is a strong indicator of how well a family functions. It also predicts children's well-being in a wide spectrum of environments and communities. Both the way that parents respond to their children and the way they direct or correct behavior are important components of good parenting. Authoritative parenting, which balances clear firm expectations for behavior with a high degree of emotional responsiveness and recognition of children's individuality, is one of the most consistent predictors of social competence from early childhood through adolescence.

Fact Or Fiction?

Spanking is effective because it stops children from misbehaving.

The Facts: While children may stop the misbehavior immediately after a spanking, experts say that it does not change future behavior. Noted development expert Penelope Leach says that when children are spanked parents may be sending the unintended message that aggression in certain circumstances is acceptable. In fact, in a longitudinal study that examined the effects of spanking, children were found to have more behavioral difficulties over time if they were spanked.

Jane Brooks, in her book *The Process of Parenting,* suggests that behavioral management techniques such as providing logical consequences, giving limited choices, and modifying the environment are more proactive and less reactive ways to guide behavior. Sharing expectations for behavior in advance of difficult situations and helping children to make better age-appropriate decisions the next time he or she faces a problem are more effective ways to coach behavior than spanking.

BEING FAIR

Fairness is a universal concern in most families. Most children know if each member is treated equally and whether everyone has the same opportunities and privileges. Rick Lavoie, a parenting expert, maintains in his frequently updated Web site that fairness in family life teaches children important lessons. He does not believe that fairness means that everyone is treated the same. He believes it is more accurate and in many cases more helpful to define fairness as everyone getting what he or she needs. His premise is that every child is unique and therefore has unique needs. The struggle for parents, according to Lavoie, is managing the inevitable conflict that treating children fairly yet differently often brings.

Q & A

Question: What are some specific rules that many families have?

Answer: Typical expectations for behavior may be negotiable, such as which coat to wear in winter. These are rules children may have input into. Other rules may not be negotiable such as wearing a coat in winter. Nonnegotiable rules often fall into two categories: those related to safety and those related to respect. Some examples of safety rules that may change with a child's age include: two-year-olds and car seat safety, 10-year-olds and bicycle safety, or 17-year-olds and driving safety. Although some rules change with age, others remain the same regardless of age. Examples of respect rules that stay the same regardless of age might be those rules related to lying or aggressive behavior.

BEING CONSISTENT

Consistency in parenting is an important element in modifying behavior. When parents want children to follow rules, it is important to enforce those rules regularly. If a particular behavior such as hitting a brother or sister is unacceptable today, it must be unacceptable tomorrow, next week, and next month. While it is nearly impossible to enforce every rule at all times, it should be parents' goal to do so. Susan M. Ward, author of *Why Consistency Is Important*, says consistency teaches children cause and effect. They learn that if they act in a certain way, there will be certain consequences. When children become capable of recognizing cause-and-effect relationships, they can begin to predict the impact of certain actions. The author and therapist Burt Segal agrees that consistency is important in establishing a trusting relationship between parent and child. He believes parents' failure to be consistent in enforcing the rules is in fact the reason why those children do not comply with those rules.

See also: Arguments and the Family; Communication Styles and Families; Family Traditions; Teens in Trouble

FURTHER READING
Brooks, Jane. *The Process of Parenting,* 7th ed. New York: McGraw-Hill, 2006.
Griffin, Lynne Reeves. *The Promise of Proactive Parenting: Sea Change.* San Diego, Calif.: Aventine Press, 2004.
Leach, Penelope. *Child Care Today: Getting It Right for Everyone.* New York: Random House, 2009.

■ FAMILY TRADITIONS

Family traditions are routines, practices, and beliefs that are passed from generation to generation. Family traditions are powerful organizers of family life. According to researcher Bobbie Crew Nelms in his 2005 article in the *Journal of Pediatric Health Care,* family traditions help to link children to other generations of the past and present. Traditions give family members a sense of security and belonging and can open up communication between individuals. Dr. Nelms describes three types of traditions: celebration traditions, such as birthdays and holidays; family traditions, which include events that the family attends together, such as a game night; and traditions that are patterned on family interactions like bedtime stories or breakfast routines.

The collection of research studies suggests that the need to bond with other family members is a universal desire among people. Dr. Vern Bengtson, professor of gerontology and sociology at the University of Southern California in Los Angeles, maintains that families provide their members with support and a sense of identity. Family members use traditions and rituals to connect with one another in positive and encouraging ways. While traditions tend to be enjoyable and family members often look forward to them, they also offer stability during difficult times and times of change.

TEENS SPEAK

Thanksgiving Dinner Is My Favorite Family Celebration

In my family, we spend Thanksgiving with my father's side of the family and Christmas Eve with my mother's. Every year both events are like small weddings with 25 to 50 people. The only thing there that seems to be more of than people are pies.

After the huge meal, all the cousins go outside to play after the huge meal. The older cousins serve as combination babysitters/team leaders in our intricate role-playing games. The farm serves as our stage to recreate favorite television shows or reenact exciting adventures. The barn is our castle, cave, or home. The farm equipment, with a little imagination, becomes racecars, boats, or space ships. I love playing these games even though many of them are too young for me now. But it's really fun to play with my younger cousins and to see them learning the games that the older cousins have been playing for years.

I love these traditions. I have such nice memories of holidays spent with my cousins. I really look forward to the next holiday, especially Thanksgiving. When I have a family of my own, I want to pass on some of these traditions to my own children.

DESCRIBING FAMILY TRADITIONS

Traditions can be described as practices in which families have engaged previously and will continue to engage. They are practices that the family values and respects. According to Susan Coady, a professor of family relations and human development at Ohio State University, traditions are characterized by predictability, regularity, and the commitment of family members. Traditions are specific to a family's cultural, religious, and racial background. Although culture, religion, or membership in a particular ethnic group might influence the occasions a family celebrates, each family individualizes the way in which it celebrates those occasions.

William Doherty, professor of family social science at the University of Minnesota, writes that family traditions are intentional ways families create patterns of connection. Doherty says that in order for a practice to truly be a family tradition, family members must be involved in the tradition in a deliberate way. The tradition must also have a special significance to family members. And to become a tradition, the practice must be repeated on a regular basis. In 2008, Dr. Doherty wrote that family is in fact the main source of information on ethics, values, and religious traditions for the child.

In a study of 28 families, Lloyd Newell found that in each family interviewed, members described a religious link to its traditions. Whether it was a faith-based holiday that brought families together or simply a set of long held beliefs or values, families made a connection between their traditions and their faith.

Fact Or Fiction?

The traditional family reunion started during medieval times in Europe.

The Facts: Family reunions are gatherings of people who descend from common ancestors. While some reunions bring together family members who simply haven't seen each other in a while, some gatherings include family members who may not know each other at all. According to researchers, such reunions originated in North America in the late 1860s. Historians believe that the reunions began in response to the traumatic family losses during the U.S. Civil War and may still be seen in African-American families as an affirmation of the end of slavery.

Family reunions became popular around the turn of the 20th century. In the 1960s, during the Vietnam War, President Lyndon B. Johnson asked Americans to hold family reunions as a way to foster national unity. Today, family reunions continue as a way to celebrate family history and draw together family members who live great distances from one another.

WHERE DO WE GO FOR THE HOLIDAYS?

Traditions, rituals, and routines can be seen in the way families celebrate holidays. According to a national poll conducted in 2001 by Harris Interactive/Modern Woodmen of America, wanting to be with family at the holidays is one of the major reasons people attend family gatherings. Celebrating religious holidays was important to 85 percent of those polled. In that same poll, 90 percent said they had attended a holiday event with family in the past three years, with 36 percent citing Thanksgiving and Christmas as the favorites.

Welcoming others into one's homes or traveling is part of the sharing of family traditions. Yet, many people claim that doing so is not easy. According to the same poll, 90 percent of Americans agree that spending time with extended family is important, but 75 percent say that getting together can be difficult.

Stressful travel is the challenge described by those who return home for the holidays. According to the American Automobile Association (AAA), more than 41 million Americans traveled 50 miles or more over the Thanksgiving weekend in 2007. Of these travelers, a little more than 33 million were traveling by car, while almost 5 million traveled by airplane and approximately 3 million people traveled by other means. For those that host or entertain family on such occasions, preparation, including cooking and cleaning, top the list of challenges to sharing family traditions.

HONORING OLD TRADITIONS

Some family traditions center on national or religious holidays. Many families also have personal practices or interpretations of their heritage and these family rituals are unique. Traditions may be written down, but more often they are passed orally from one generation to the next.

Many traditions have evolved from cultural, religious, and recreational activities that families have adopted over the years. Some family traditions celebrate the past and connect family members to their roots. Honoring old traditions, experts say, builds a shared understanding of family heritage and a sense of community. Sharing unique memories and reflections is an important part of family life.

Traditions are also important because they keep the generations in contact with one another. In a 2008 study, the researchers Casey Copen and Merril Silverstein looked at the effect of multigenerational influence on traditions and religious beliefs. They write that grandparents play an important role in the lives of their grandchildren and that they help to shape children's religious beliefs, values, and practices. The authors explain that as grandparents share stories with their grandchildren, they are also imparting family history and traditions.

CELEBRATING NEW TRADITIONS

As families change, traditions change. As new family members are added through marriage and the birth of children, the dynamic of family life changes. In the early years of a new marriage, couples begin to sort through the traditions that each has brought from his or her family of origin. Together, they begin to examine their individual family histories and negotiate what their new traditions will be.

Traditions are important to families with young children, because the parents are at a stage in life when they want to establish their own traditions and perhaps break away from those of previous generations. For example, when children begin to anticipate the traditions of Christmas, their parents may prefer to celebrate Christmas in their own home instead of traveling to their parents' homes.

More often than not, traditions within a family evolve slowly over time into new traditions with few, if any, dramatic breaks with the past. Yet even small alterations in the rituals and routines of family holidays or activities may lead to significant changes in traditions.

Q & A

Question: What is meant by "rites of passage"?

Answer: Rites of passage are ceremonies or observances associated with the transition from one place or stage of life to another. Rites of passage may be formal, such as the Jewish ritual called a bar mitzvah or bat mitzvah. It signifies the beginning of a boy or girl assuming adult responsibilities in Judaism. Other rites of passage are informal, such as the recognition that a child may be old enough to have a later bedtime or learn to drive a car. Rites of passage, when celebrated or acknowledged, help children and adults understand and respect the responsibilities and privileges that come from moving to a new developmental stage.

INCLUDING RELATIVES IN TRADITIONS

At the core of the celebration of family traditions is the desire to include treasured friends and relatives. Numerous family customs include aunts, uncles, and other extended family members and special guests.

While many families look forward to time spent together, for some family members, time spent with relatives can be challenging. The Mayo Clinic says that distance, extended family obligations, finances, work responsibilities, health concerns, scheduling conflicts, religious differences, and personality issues may contribute to the high levels of stress some family members may experience when they participate in family traditions. Honest, open communication and compromises, experts say, are the key to keeping healthy family traditions alive and enjoyable.

Given the strength that family traditions bring to family life, Susan A. Lieberman of Rice University in Houston, Texas, believes that families today need tradition now more than ever before. "The world is changing so rapidly now, and traditions give us an anchor. Traditions make you feel good as a family. These indelible memories bring character and texture to our lives."

See also: Birth Order and Psychology; Death in the Family; Family Rules; Religion and the Family; The Traditional Family

FURTHER READING

Atlas, Nava. *Everyday Traditions: Simple Family Rituals for Connection and Comfort.* Poughkeepsie, N.Y.: Amberwood Press, 2005.

Coleman, Marilyn, Lawrence H. Ganong, and Kelly Warzinik. *Family Life in Twentieth-Century America.* Santa Barbara, Calif.: Greenwood Publishing Group, 2007.

Doherty, William. *The Intentional Family: How to Build Family Ties in Our Modern World.* New York: Avon Books, 1999.

Pleck, Elizabeth Hafkin. *Celebrating the Family: Ethnicity, Consumer Culture, and Family Rituals.* Cambridge, Mass.: Harvard University Press, 2000.

■ FINANCIAL MANAGEMENT, MARITAL

Marital financial management involves the organization of a family's money, property, and other wealth. When a couple marries, they make a financial and legal commitment to one another. The couple shares the financial and legal benefits of the union. Those benefits may include being entitled to one another's work benefits such as health insurance and pension. Good financial management requires two people willing to learn about finances and to be responsible with money.

Some couples draw up a **prenuptial agreement** prior to marriage. It is a legal agreement arranged before marriage stating who owns property acquired before marriage and during the marriage and how property will be divided in the event of divorce. Many couples prepare **wills.** These legal documents express a person's wishes regarding the disposal of his or her property after death. In the event of an emergency, a husband and wife are often encouraged to keep good records regarding their finances and provide one another with **power of attorney.** A power of attorney is a legal document that authorizes another person to act on one's behalf. Other financial management considerations in marriage include the process of changing one's name, opening bank accounts, paying family bills, acquiring stocks and bonds, and managing debt and credit cards.

PRENUPTIAL AGREEMENTS

Some couples, prior to marriage, draw up a contract detailing what each is bringing to the marriage and how, in the event of one's death, these **assets** are to be distributed. Such agreements protect funds each individual had prior to the marriage. While most couples enter into a prenuptial agreement to protect separate property and money, some couples enter into one to protect themselves from each other's **debt.** According to Lee Borden, a noted lawyer specializing in these arrangements, remarriage, blending families, and high divorce rates are the reasons some couples feel more financially secure entering into a marriage with a prenuptial agreement.

WILLS

A will is a legal document stating what should happen to the money, property, and belongings of a person after his or her death. A will shows how to distribute the property of the deceased, and how children of the deceased will be provided for. As assets grow during a marriage and the family expands and changes, couples are encouraged to review their wills from time to time to see if alterations need to be made.

TAX BENEFITS

Income tax is a tax on earnings payable to city, state, and/or federal governments. Married couples may file tax returns separately or together. Many couples enjoy tax benefits when filing returns jointly. The way a couple is taxed differs from the way a single person is taxed. In most cases, couples save money by filing tax returns together. Another benefit of filing a joint return is the **tax credits** that are offered to married couples. However, if couples file taxes together, they are responsible for one another. If one spouse doesn't pay what is owed, the other spouse must pay for both.

INSURANCE BENEFITS

Life insurance is paid to a stated family member in the event of the death of the person insured. Most state laws allow a spouse a portion of the benefits from a spouse's life insurance policy, even if the policy was purchased prior to the marriage. These laws are complex, yet often they override the recipient actually named in the policy, paying some, if not all, monies to the surviving spouse.

Some couples make sure that they each carry enough life insurance during their marriage to handle potentially difficult financial situations that may result from the death of one spouse. Many purchase policies large enough to pay a mortgage or provide day care for young children in the event of either spouse's death.

SOCIAL SECURITY BENEFITS

Monthly benefits are paid to eligible people from a federal government agency called the Social Security Administration. Those that are eligible include individuals over the age of 66 who have worked for ten years or more and paid into the Social Security system, their spouses, and dependent children as well as disabled persons of any age. The rules and regulations are complex. Yet, it is an important benefit that married couples can share if eligibility criteria are met.

DID YOU KNOW?

Legal Documents for Unmarried Couples

Did you know that unmarried couples can obtain some of the rights of married couples by arranging for certain legal documents? Among the documents that may afford unmarried couples similar rights as married couples are the following:

Power of Attorney for Health Care Decisions
Power of Attorney for Financial Decisions
Living Together Agreement
Will

Source: Alternatives to Marriage Project, Albany, NY: 2004.

Couples can also receive veteran and military benefits, including special loans. Such benefits may be used to pay living expenses, help pay for education, or medical care.

PENSIONS

A pension is income paid after retirement. Some companies offer their employees pension plans so that when workers retire they receive a monthly income. A number of large companies offer **profit sharing.** Profit sharing is a plan in which employers share their profits with employees at the employer's discretion. The compensation may be stocks, bonds, or cash and can be paid immediately or deferred until retirement. According to Christian Weller of the Center for American Progress, a nonprofit financial information organization, only 43.2 percent of private sector employees had an employer-sponsored retirement plan in 2006. Many people today purchase private pension plans. These plans play an important financial role for couples in planning for retirement.

PROPERTY

Property that is obtained by either spouse individually or the couple together during a marriage is considered marital property. The time frame starts the day the couple marries and lasts until the date that the couple begins to live apart. Nine states are known as **community** property states: Arizona, California, Idaho, Louisiana, Nevada, New Mexico, Texas, Washington, and Wisconsin. The Commonwealth of Puerto Rico is also a community property jurisdiction. In each of these places, all property obtained during the marriage—other than a gift or inheritance—belongs equally to each spouse. Even if one spouse earned all of the money used to obtain the property, the government views the property as belonging to both parties. While these laws differ, each is based on the idea that both spouses contribute equally to the marriage and therefore all property obtained during the marriage is the result of their combined efforts.

Each person owns the property he or she brought to the marriage separately, unless the owner wants the property to be jointly owned. Lawyers can help couples clarify arrangements so that in case of death, it is clear which property is separately owned and which is jointly owned.

WORKER'S COMPENSATION

Worker's compensation is a payment received for injury on the job. This state-governed system addresses injuries that are work-related. Under the system, employers pay the cost of medical treatment and lost pay that results from a worker's job-related injury or disease, regardless of who is at fault. In return, the employee gives up the right to sue the employer, even if the injuries are due to carelessness on the employer's part.

If a person receiving worker's compensation dies, his or her spouse is due the worker's compensation benefits owed to the deceased.

NEXT-OF-KIN PRIVILEGES

The term next-of-kin refers to a person's closest living relative either by blood or by marriage. In marriage, the term has legal significance. It has become a term that describes those individuals who are most closely related to the deceased and therefore eligible to inherit his or her money and property. Laws have been established to clarify the rights of a person's next-of-kin.

Some next-of-kin privileges relate to visitation when the individual is ill or hospitalized. For example, the wife of a terminally ill man can remain with him in intensive care at the hospital. She is allowed to make medical decisions regarding his care when he is no longer able to make these decisions. The hospital will follow her instructions for the after-death procedures, and she has the authority to make burial arrangements. Visitation of a relative convicted of a crime and sent to prison is also covered in next-of-kin privileges.

RECORD KEEPING

Keeping financial information organized and accessible is an important aspect of financial management. Some couples use files for most papers and safe deposit boxes held at a bank for particularly important papers. Documents that require safekeeping include the marriage certificate, car titles, proof of property held prior to marriage, social security cards, canceled checks, birth certificates, adoption records, credit card charge slips, copies of tax returns, insurance policies, property deeds, stocks and bonds, military discharge papers, veteran's benefits, death certificates of family members, divorce and custody agreements, passports, and children's immunization records. Couples sometimes keep copies of these documents in more than one separate location in case of fire.

Q & A

Question: If one spouse is responsible for paying all the bills each month, how will the other spouse know the couple's financial situation?

Answer: Early in a marriage, experts recommend coming up with a system for paying bills and another system for communicating the family's financial picture to one another. Financial experts recommend regular discussions about current finances as well as regular discussions about financial goals.

OTHER FINANCIAL CONCERNS

Changing a name

Many women change their last names to the last name of the person they are marrying, while others prefer to keep their maiden or family name. Legally speaking, either decision is acceptable. Whether a name is changed or not, it is best for women to sign all papers during the marriage with only one name.

Assets

Stocks and bonds purchased before the marriage are not community property unless the person wishes to have them be jointly owned. Many people have separate bank accounts prior to marriage but open a joint account when they marry. Whether or not couples maintain separate accounts or opt for a joint account is a matter of personal preference. Yet, once couples deposit money into a joint account, the money becomes the property of both people.

Debt and credit cards

Before a couple marries, each may have his or her own credit report. Regardless of how good either party's credit rating, it does not affect anyone else's rating. However, when a couple marries and tries to secure a loan to buy a house or other property, the bank will look at both ratings. Partners who live in a community property state find that all of the debts one spouse may incur during their marriage are considered the other spouse's debts as well. For example, if one spouse buys a car and then doesn't keep up the payments, the bank can make the other spouse pay for the car. If one spouse applies for credit, the other spouse's debts may hinder his or her chances of receiving credit.

Financial advisers strongly suggest that before couples marry, they discuss how they will handle their finances during their marriage. They should consider how they will divide expenses, make purchases, and manage long term financial planning.

Given the complexity of financial management, it's easy to see why many couples disagree about money. Ruth Hayden, a financial educator, offers practical methods for financial management for couples. Hayden suggests that spouses meet each other halfway, with feet firmly planted in security while still stretching to make compromises. Frequent communication and the setting of financial goals are the key to a strong financial plan, Hayden says.

Fact Or Fiction?

A person needn't be concerned with financial management in marriage until he or she is an adult.

The Facts: Managing money is a skill that can be learned. Experts say that early positive experiences in managing money provide a strong foundation for managing money later in life. Teens can learn about managing money by watching the way in which the people around them manage money. Observing how parents spend and save teaches teens valuable lessons. When teens manage small amounts of their own money, they also learn important lessons on the value of managing money well as well as the consequence of various spending decisions.

Child support

Every parent has a legal requirement to support his or her children. Money paid by a parent to help support children who are not living with him or her is called **child support**. Child support can be paid voluntarily or be ordered by a court. The support may come in different forms including a one-time payment, regular installments paid directly to the custodial parent, or regular deductions from a paycheck paid directly to the custodial parent. Child support can be costly and may create conflict between parents caring for children but living apart.

Power of attorney

If one spouse becomes too ill to manage legal and financial matters the other spouse may need to have the legal right to manage the household. But to do so, the spouse may need a document called a "power of attorney." For example, if a person needs to sell a car that is jointly owned and his or her spouse is seriously ill, then this document provides a way to make the sale. Many couples who are facing the onset of a serious illness get legal assistance in drawing up a power-of-attorney document.

Health insurance

Families vary in the way they handle health insurance. In some families, one person will carry the medical coverage for the entire family through his or her employer. Not all employers offer insurance and both spouses may not work. So, this decision is often based on the type and cost of coverage offered by the employers of the working spouse or spouses.

Financial management in marriage is complex. The more a couple learns and plans together for a strong financial future, the more they can enjoy the financial and legal benefits of their marital status.

When managing finances, couples may benefit from keeping good records, reading about financial planning and obtaining the support of professionals in financial management and the law.

See also: Arguments and the Family; Day Care; Death in the Family; Family Counseling; Gay Parents; Single-Parent Families

FURTHER READING
Bach, David. *Smart Couples Finish Rich.* New York: Broadway Books, 2002.

Barnhill, Julie. *Til Debt Do Us Part*. Eugene, Oreg.: Harvest House Publishers, 2002.

Hall, Fiona. *How to Set up a Family Budget*. Scotts Valley, Calif.: CreateSpace, 2010.

Inglesias, Robinson. *Money Matters: A Common Sense Guide to Financial Nourishment*. Bloomington, Ind.: iUniverse Inc., 2005.

Wagner, Michael J. *Your Money, Day One: How to Start Right and End Rich*. Charleston, S.C.: BookSurge Publishing, 2009.

■ GAY PARENTS

Gay parents are those who are **homosexual** in their sexual orientation—that is, they are attracted to people of the same sex. **Sexual orientation** refers to one's enduring romantic, emotional, or sexual attraction to a person of the opposite sex and/or one's own sex. People who are **heterosexual** are attracted to the opposite sex. People with a homosexual orientation are referred to as gay (both men and women) or lesbian (women only). A person who is **bisexual** is attracted to both men and women. A person who is **transsexual** has an overwhelming desire to live his or her life as a member of the opposite sex. Bisexual and transsexual persons can also be parents. Their issues are similar to those of gay parents and are often discussed together.

The concept of sexual orientation refers to more than sexual behavior. It includes the way in which a person describes his or her identity. Some individuals may identify themselves as gay, lesbian, or bisexual without engaging in any sexual activity. Individuals may become aware at different points in their lives that they are heterosexual, gay, lesbian, bisexual, or transsexual.

According to the U.S. census, many gay couples have children and research shows that these families have much in common with other families. Yet, gay families still face discrimination by those who believe that exposure to gay men and women will in some way harm a child's development.

CHILDREN IN GAY PARTNERSHIPS

The number of gay parents in the United States has been previously estimated to be around 5 million to 6 million. However, according to the researcher Jamie Landou, gay and lesbian parenting has increased. In fact, the 2010 U.S. Census includes questions to encourage the reporting of same-sex couples and same-sex parents in a household. This new opportunity for research will yield a more accurate depiction of the makeup of American families.

The majority of gay parents had their children in a heterosexual relationship. Following divorce or separation they entered into a gay partnership and their children from the previous relationship were included in their new family. In other families, one or both gay parents have adopted the children. Some lesbians have children through **artificial insemination** (the placement of sperm into a female reproductive tract by means other than sexual intercourse). According to an article in the journal *Pediatrics,* the researcher J. G. Pawelski estimates that, as of 2006, 10 million U.S. schoolchildren have lesbian, gay, bisexual, or transgendered parents. For lesbian and gay parents, there are many ways to create a family. According to Cynthia Telingator, M.D., and Charlotte Patterson, Ph.D., lesbian and gay parents might have a child from a previous heterosexual relationship or marriage, through a pregnancy from biological conception or artificial insemination, working with a surrogate, or through adoption or being a foster parent.

Dr. Telingator and Dr. Patterson also found that children of same-sex parents reported the same levels of anxiety, self-esteem, grade point averages, graduation rates, and peer relationships as compared to children of other-sex parents. The research concludes that the gender of a child's parents is not an indicator as to the health and well-being of the child. Also, while the authors contend that living with same-sex parents may present challenges in facing some discrimination, these challenges have not been shown to harm the overall health of the child. Instead, for all children and teens, no matter the gender of their parents, the quality of family relationships is more important in determining the satisfaction levels of children.

The American Psychological Association (APA) has been researching the effects of lesbian and gay parenting on children since the 1970s. The APA asserts that the sexual and gender identities of children of lesbian and gay parents, such as their gender-role behavior and sexual orientation, do not develop differently than those of children from other-sex parents. In fact, the APA notes that many concerns voiced over lesbian and gay parenting are rooted in prejudice and lack of education instead of facts and proven research. The organization contends that the development, adjustment, and well-being of the children of gay or lesbian parents are no different than the children of heterosexual parents. Research suggests that children of gay parents have normal relationships with friends and that their relationships with adults of both sexes are also satisfactory.

Dr. Charlotte Patterson, following extensive research on children of gay parents, has found that these children experience the same concerns and problems during a divorce as do their heterosexual family counterparts. Other studies confirm those findings. When examining the causes for emotional or behavior problems in children, many researchers find the problems stem from such factors as parents' depression, custody battles, or other conflicts between divorcing or separating parents. The connection between being raised by gay parents and an increase in emotional and behavioral problems in children is not supported by current research.

Fact Or Fiction?

Children raised with gay parents are more likely to become gay adults.

The Facts: Research to date shows that children raised by gay and lesbian parents are no more likely to become homosexual than children raised by heterosexuals. In general, the studies suggest that when children of gay parents become young adults, they are more likely to have had or considered same-sex relationships but are no more likely than children of straight parents to identify themselves as lesbian, gay, or bisexual.

A variety of studies reveal that the percentage of children of gay parents who have a homosexual orientation is equivalent to a random sample of the general population. A review of studies assessing 300 children born to gay or lesbian parents in 12 different samples shows no evidence of any disturbances in the development of sexual identity among those studied.

SOCIETAL REACTIONS

Numerous public opinion polls over the past 25 years indicate that attitudes toward gay men, lesbians, and bisexuals have become more positive. Yet compared to other social groups, gay families still experience discrimination in all aspects of daily life. More recently several states have recognized the rights of gay people to employment free of discrimination but there are no federal laws prohibiting discrimination against homosexuals in employment, housing, military service, and public accommodations. Groups representing the rights of gay people such as the American Civil Liberties Union are presenting their case to the federal government about the need to provide the same civil rights protections to gay people that are afforded to racial minorities, women, the disabled, and the elderly. While more laws at the state and federal level will continue to be proposed and passed, one major accomplishment in providing equal protection to gay individuals was the passing in 2009 of the federal Hate Crimes Prevention Act (IICPA). This law allows the Department of Justice to investigate and prosecute crimes in which a victim has been targeted due to his or her actual or perceived race, color, religion, national origin, gender, sexual orientation or gender identity, or disability status.

Gay parents and their children sometimes experience prejudice and isolation from other family members, neighbors, employers, and society in general. Psychologists from Loyola Marymount University published an article in response to the need for more programming for lesbian, gay, bisexual, transgender, and questioning (LGBTQ) youth in academic settings. The authors wrote that many LGBTQ students are at a greater risk for harassment and victimization as a result of discrimination. They illustrated the need for teachers, school psychologists, administrators, and counselors to work together in creating a safe environment that leads to academic success and positive emotional development. Currently, many schools are creating programs to address the specific concerns and needs of the LGBTQ student body.

However, young people and children are not the only ones who face challenges. The University of Florida researchers Dana Berkowitz and William Marsiglio explain that society views parenthood and heterosexuality as so synonymous that the idea of homosexual parents can be viewed as a shock to the system. They write that American culture also tends to give more attention to mothers, thus creating more challenges for gay men who have a child than for lesbians who choose to create a family.

TEENS SPEAK

My Parents Are Gay

I found out my parents were gay when I was seven. Up until then, I just thought families had two dads, two moms, or one of each. I just didn't give it that much thought. But when I came home from school and asked my dad what "gay" meant, he sat me down and told me. At first, I thought maybe it was bad to have gay parents. Kids teased me and my dads always asked me if I was okay about that. With so much attention being paid to it, I started to think maybe something was wrong with it. Now that I am a teenager, I know that lots of people are really uncomfortable with this subject and even mean and judgmental. But I still don't really see why people are having so much trouble understanding that when two people love each other, they just want to be a family. Why people judge other people is just something I don't think I will ever understand. My parents are my parents; I love them just as much as anyone else loves their parents.

LEGAL AND FINANCIAL IMPLICATIONS

In almost every state, gay people cannot legally marry one another. In some, they cannot adopt children or become foster parents. Those who already have children may face restrictions related to custody of their children or visitation rights. Because a homosexual relationship is not recognized as a marriage by the federal government or most state governments, gay parents often draw up legal documents to protect a partner's right to inherit property, participate in medical decision making, and assume guardianship of the children.

Without legal protections, gay parents and their children may find themselves unable to claim such benefits as life insurance, Social Security, or an inheritance if a parent dies.

According to the Services and Advocacy for Gay, Lesbian, Bisexual, or Transgender Elders, or SAGE, the world's oldest and largest non-profit organization designed to assist gay, lesbian, bisexual, and transgender (GLBT) seniors, there are more than 2 million GLBT elders in the United States. In the publication *Outing Age 2010,* SAGE addressed several issues that GLBT seniors face. For one, financial benefits such as Social Security are not awarded to a GLBT senior's partner when he or she passes away, as they are in heterosexual marriages. Also, many GLBT seniors live alone. The older GLBT community faces different challenges than the younger generations. Because of this, more researchers and organizations that study aging are getting involved. For example, the American Society for Aging and the AARP (formerly the American Association of Retired Persons) are now working with the SAGE organization to focus on the specific vulnerabilities of GLBT seniors.

CULTURAL AND RELIGIOUS ISSUES

Even as research and public opinion polls show an overall rise in acceptance of gay men and women, many Americans are opposed to homosexual behaviors. Numerous studies have been conducted by Gregory M. Herek, a professor of psychology at the University of California at Davis, on changing attitudes toward gay people. While the overall attitude toward gay people has become more favorable, when it comes to religion and homosexuality, attitudes remain unfavorable.

As he published in the *Journal of Social Issues* and other journals in 2007, the researcher G. M. Herek found that although acceptance of homosexuality has been improving in many areas, discrimination remains very strong in certain sectors of American society. He explains that while religion is one of these areas, so is law and medicine. Originally, homosexuality was looked down upon as part of the broader topic of sexual conduct not intending procreation. While many religious organizations choose to avoid the topic of homosexuality, others choose to make a public statement condemning it.

For instance, while the Roman Catholic Church states that homosexual acts are wrong, the church also condemns any discrimination against gay and lesbian members, especially those who do not act on their homosexuality. This supports an older, many feel hypocritical school of thought, that being gay is not a sin, but acting upon it is. For other churches, such as the Presbyterian Church and the United Methodist Church, gay members are encouraged to attend; however, they cannot hold official positions within the church. In still other denominations, not only are gay members allowed to practice but they also may be ordained as ministers.

Therefore, even with religious opposition, attitudes about gay relationships are changing even in faith-based communities. With the numbers of gay couples parenting on the rise, social and religious debate over gay marriage and parenting will surely continue. And while some people feel or believe that children in families with gay parents are disadvantaged in some way, this view is not supported by current research.

Q & A

Question: What are some positive attributes found in children who grow up with gay parents?

Answer: While there are advantages and disadvantages to growing up in all types of families, the researcher Richard Redding at Duke University has found some specific attributes in the children of gay parents. For instance, because it is impossible for two same-sex parents to naturally conceive a child, almost all children born to a gay couple are planned, in comparison to the sometimes unwanted pregnancies that can occur in heterosexual relationships. Also, some research suggests that children of same-sex parents grow to be more tolerant and accepting of others, which may come from their own experiences with real or perceived discrimination. However, these important values can be taught to children of any family makeup.

See also: Adoption; Family, The New; Marriage and Family, Change In; Religion and the Family

FURTHER READING

Drucker, Jane, and Harold Schulweis. *Lesbian and Gay Families Speak Out: Understanding the Joys and Challenges of Diverse Family Life.* Boulder, Colo.: Perseus Publishing, 2001.

Fakhrid-Deen, Tina. *Let's Get This Straight: The Ultimate Handbook for Youth with LGBTQ Parents.* Berkeley, Calif.: Seal Press, 2010.

Fields, Julianna. *Gay and Lesbian Parents: The Changing Face of Modern Families.* Broomall, Pa.: Mason Crest Publishers, 2009.

Garner, Abigail. *Families Like Mine: Children of Gay Parents Tell It Like It Is.* New York: HarperCollins, 2004.

Johnson, Suzanne M., and Elizabeth O'Connor. *The Gay Baby Boom: The Psychology of Gay Parenthood.* New York: New York University Press, 2002.

Kenrick, Joanna. *Out.* (gr8reads). Edinburgh, Scotland: Barrington Stoke Ltd, 2010.

■ INDEPENDENCE

In this case, the desire to break away from parents and create one's own set of values. With the onset of puberty, among the many emotional changes on the road to adulthood are adolescents' yearnings to be different from their parents. When Mom or Dad makes a request or a demand, it might cause more friction than it used to. Because adolescents are struggling with newfound sexuality, they want more privacy. Friends, music, clothes—all take on a new importance as a young person begins to explore identity and self-expression. A gap often begins to widen between parent and child and the experiences of each, and the child will often respond by wanting to make more decisions alone.

Seeking independence is a healthy and necessary part of becoming an adult, but perhaps no other single factor about the transition from childhood to adulthood creates more stress for parents and children alike. Sometimes parents react by becoming less patient and more controlling; sometimes their children become rebellious and disrespectful. In both cases, each is reacting to the changes and their own discomfort with the new conflicts they create. Admittedly, it can be a frightening time for all.

TEENS SPEAK

You Can Trust Me

My dad doesn't trust me. Not one bit. Every time I leave the house, he wants to know where I'm going, who I'm going to be with, what adult will be around to keep an eye on us, and when I'll be home. I feel like a criminal having to check in with a parole officer. I mean, I'm 13 years old—why can't he just trust me?

It was better before last summer, when I was hanging around with Evan, a kid from the neighborhood who is a little older than me. Evan had just gotten a pellet gun for his birthday, and he was letting me shoot it. One of the pellets bounced off the metal target and broke a window in a neighbor's house, and when the neighbor yelled at Evan, he swore at him. Then the neighbor called the police.

I got in trouble even though I didn't even shoot the pellet gun (at least not that time), and I didn't say a word to the neighbor. The cops talked to my dad; he got mad, but not real mad, especially after I told him what happened. But after that, every time I go outside, he started asking me all these questions.

I stopped hanging around with Evan after that anyway. To tell you the truth, he's kind of a bully and not a lot of fun to hang around with anyway. I've got some new friends now, and my dad told me he wants to meet them. They're coming over tomorrow to play soccer in the backyard. My dad said he might play too, which would be cool.

HEALTHY INDEPENDENCE

In every person's life, there comes a time when independence is necessary. How soon should a teenager have the chance to test the waters? Is it ever truly "safe" to do so?

Teenagers should first understand that parents are rarely eager to let go: It goes against our instinctual nature to protect our young. However, even parents understand that the time will come when they must allow their child to begin to live and grow on their own. The problem is, for parents, that time always feels like it comes too soon.

The truth is that it can be very difficult to figure out how much independence is good and how much is dangerous. At the same time, allowing too little independence can be a bad thing too; it can cause a person to be too sheltered or it can provoke some teenagers into breaking rules that they find too restrictive. What makes it even more difficult is the fact that because every child is different, there is really no simple schedule to follow when beginning to grant a little freedom. What is appropriate for one 13-year-old might be completely wrong for the next. (That, of course, makes things very difficult when you are talking about two 13-year-old friends.)

As with so many other transitions during young adulthood, the solution to this conflict is found in communication. It is important not to make demands, but it is perfectly healthy to talk with your parents about—even suggest—reasonable ways you might be given more independence. Also, remember that independence is usually earned, just like the trust that comes with it.

Matt Sanders, a professor of clinical psychology in New Zealand and a parenting expert, suggests that parents and children start small. Perhaps a teenager will have more freedom to decide how to spend an allowance, a birthday gift of cash, or other pocket money. The teenager might be allowed to choose a gift for a friend or family member or to make up the guest list for a party without a parent's input. Even when it comes to chores and homework, the student can start to take more responsibility to decide when and how the tasks are completed, rather than being told how to do them.

Small bits of independence will do two things: It will allow trust to develop between the parents and child and it will begin to give the teenager a taste of freedom and the responsibility that comes with it. Rather than running to adults to solve problems, although they might provide important input to help you make decisions, many decisions are now yours to make. Make them carefully and try to learn from your mistakes as these early experiences will be the best learning experiences you likely will have, painful as they sometimes might be.

Q & A

Question: What's an easy way to show my parents I can handle a little more independence?

Answer: Get involved in youth activities or sports in your school or community. You can learn a great many new skills, and most of them will be skills you can use at home. There will be a level of responsibility—for attending practices, rehearsals, or meetings—and as you have some success, your parents will start to see you in a new way. As a result, they might begin to allow you a little more independence. When that happens, be sure to *follow through,* because it is much harder to win back confidence after you lose it.

HOW MUCH IS TOO MUCH?

It is important to remember that freedom is never absolute. There are always rules to follow.

First, there are areas where parents have every right to know what you are doing and to maintain some control until you reach adulthood: when you are home at night, where you are going, whom you are going with, what movies you see, and how you are doing in school. Even when a teenager achieves some independence, these are areas in which young people have an obligation to include their parents—and to honor the rules they set.

Also, although it can be difficult for teenagers to acknowledge, they still have a great deal to learn about the world. They will only learn by making mistakes, but sometimes those mistakes carry devastating consequences, and parents correctly want to protect their teens from those consequences. When parents begin to pull back a little, try to understand why: Very often, it truly is for your own good. Part of independence, by the way, is understanding that disagreements occur and a different opinion must be respected and, in the case of parents, accepted. Your health and safety have to come first.

Fact Or Fiction?

Most parents are okay with letting their sons and daughters date before age 16.

The Facts: In a recent survey by International Communications Research of teenagers age 12 to 17 and their parents, 87 percent of parents said teens should be at least age 16 before they begin steady, one-on-one dating. Almost half of the teenagers agreed. The older the teenager surveyed, the more likely they are to say that steady dating should be delayed until at least age 16—suggesting that experience leads them to believe early dating is a bad idea.

Freedom has four parts

The psychologist Dr. Carl Pickhardt suggests in a June 2009 article in *Psychology Today* that independence involves four components: responsibility, accountability, work, and self-help. Parents have a role in each of those. They should make sure a young person is "taking care of business at home, at school, and out in the world before consenting to any new degree of freedom that is desired." They can teach accountability by making sure the teenager understands the consequences that come from having the power to make decisions and that the teenager deals with the consequences. They can help a child learn how important the time and effort invested can be in reaching goals. Finally, parents need to let children learn a lot of this on their own, ensuring the lessons will last a lifetime.

Teenagers have a role in that as well—helping their parents understand that a healthy balance of independence and support will be a safe way to try the real world of adulthood, both good and bad.

See also: Arguments and the Family; Family, The New; Family, The Traditional; Family Rules; Religion and the Family; Teens in Trouble

FURTHER READING

Bachel, Beverly K. *What Do You Really Want? How to Set a Goal and Go for It! A Guide for Teens.* Minneapolis, Minn.: Free Spirit Publishing, 2001.

Covey, Sean. *The 6 Most Important Decisions You'll Ever Make: A Guide for Teens.* Whitby, Ontario, Canada: Fireside Publishing, 2006.

Pelzer, Dave. *Help Yourself for Teens: Real-Life Advice for Real-Life Challenges.* New York: Plume Books, 2005.

■ MARRIAGE AND FAMILY, CHANGES IN

Both men and women today are marrying later in life than at any other time in the past 100 years. Changing beliefs about appropriate family roles have led to greater sharing of household and economic responsibilities. These changes in marriage and family have occurred largely in response to economic and cultural pressures.

DOMESTIC PARTNERS

According to the census of 2009, 6.6 million unmarried couples were cohabiting—that is, living together. In 1960, the census reported that fewer than 500,000 unmarried couples were living together. About 60 percent of those couples were between 25 and 44 years of age and 36 percent had children under the age of 15. According to the U.S. Census Bureau, many couples live together before marrying. In 2000, more than half of heterosexual couples who planned to marry cohabited before they were wed. In 1965, that figure was 10 percent. Despite fierce opposition to cohabitation by religious and conservative groups, an increasing number of unmarried couples are living together, either as a prelude to marriage or because of a lifestyle choice.

People cohabit for many reasons. It may be a utilitarian arrangement in which partners live together to share costs and household tasks. They may or may not have an intimate relationship with their housemate. Other couples see cohabitation as a trial marriage, a chance to test their compatibility and decide if they want to marry. Couples who are planning to marry may move in together during the engagement period, often because they see no reason to live apart while preparing for a wedding.

Some cohabiting couples who are intimately involved engage in sex only with each other. They have a **monogamous** relationship. These couples may view cohabitation as a substitute for marriage and do not intend to marry for practical or philosophical reasons. For instance, marriage may mean the loss of financial benefits such as financial support from a former spouse (alimony) or a former employer (pension payments). One or both of the partners may be separated but not divorced from a previous marriage or have been unhappily married in the past and not wish to marry again. In most states, cohabitation is the only option available to same-sex couples. However, most cohabitating couples are heterosexual.

Fact Or Fiction?

Families are becoming a thing of the past.

The Facts: Although the divorce rate remains high, and the percentage of unmarried couples who live together has climbed in recent years, there is no evidence that Americans are giving up on marriage or families. Most people who cohabitate eventually marry, and most people who divorce remarry within a few years of their divorce. While this trend helps to create blended families and other complex family structures, it does not seem to indicate that marriage as an institution is about to dissolve. Americans still want to marry. But they also want the freedom to leave marriages that are not happy. Instead of spending a lifetime in an unhappy marriage, Americans are ending unfulfilling marital partnerships and searching for better marriages and happier family lives.

The rapid increase in the number of cohabitating couples in the United States has prompted some employers and some local governments to recognize these couples as **domestic partners.** While definitions of domestic partnership vary widely, it is usually defined as a stable, intimate relationship between two people who are financially interdependent. Employers may offer domestic partners the same benefit plans, including health insurance, provided to married employees. Some city and state governments also recognize domestic partnerships. Legal status as domestic partners may or may not result in tangible benefits, such as shared health insurance plans.

Within one and one-half years of moving in together, half of cohabiting couples either marry or break up. Domestic partnerships may be less stable than marriages, according to a 2000 study released by the Centers for Disease Control and Prevention (CDC). CDC researchers found that the probability of a cohabitation breaking up within five years is 49 percent compared to the 20 percent chance of a first marriage ending in divorce within five years. After 10 years, the chance that a first marriage will end is 33 percent compared with 62 percent for cohabitation. In general, unmarried couples who live together report poorer relationships than their married counterparts. In 2002, 34.5 percent of domestic partnerships versus 18.7 percent of marriages were dissolved. CDC researchers speculate that the poorer quality reported by cohabitating couples could be due to less commitment to a lasting partnership.

However, the unions of domestic partners who plan to marry do not appear to be significantly different from those who wait until marriage to live together. While some studies have suggested a link between cohabitation before marriage and an increased risk of divorce, a 2003 study by Jay Teachman, a sociologist at Western Washington University, challenges this theory. Teachman asked women who participated in the 1995 National Survey of Family Growth whether they had engaged in premarital sex and cohabitation before marriage. He found no link between divorce and premarital sex, and divorce and cohabitation for women who eventually married their domestic partner. His research suggests that women who are committed to a single relationship do not increase their risk of divorce.

DELAYED MARRIAGE

Both men and women in the United States are waiting longer to marry. In 1890, the median age at first marriage was 26 years for men and 22 years for women. For most of the early 20th century, the age at which people wed decreased steadily, reaching a low of 22.5 years for men and 20.1 years for women in the mid-1950s. By 1959, nearly half of all women were under the age of 19 when they married.

Historian Steven Mintz, a professor at the University of Houston, attributes the decline in age at first marriage during the early 1900s to economic and social factors. As more people left farms to work in cities and towns, a new idea about marriage developed: the **companionate family**, one in which the family is seen as the primary source of emotional satisfaction and personal happiness. These two influences

Median Age at First Marriage, 1890–2008

Median Age at First Marriage of the Population 15 Years and Over by Sex: Selected Years, 1890 to 2008.

Year	Males	Females
1890	26.1	22.0
1900	25.9	21.9
1910	25.1	21.6
1920	24.6	21.2
1930	24.3	21.3
1940	24.3	21.5
1950	22.8	20.3
1960	22.8	20.3
1970	23.2	20.8
1980	24.7	22.0
1990	26.1	23.9
1993	26.5	24.5
1994	26.7	24.5
1995	26.9	24.5
1996	27.1	24.8
1997	26.8	25.0
1998	26.7	25.0
1999	26.9	25.1
2000	26.8	25.1
2001	26.9	25.1
2002	26.9	25.3
2003	27.1	25.3
2005	27.0	25.5
2006	27.5	25.9
2007	27.7	26.0
2008	27.6	25.9

Source: U.S. Census Bureau.

combined to lead many couples to marry as a way to escape the social isolation of the city, seeking intimacy and fulfillment from marriage and early childbearing.

Age at first marriage increased slightly during the 1930s—a period of much poverty and unemployment across the nation. Marriages were postponed as people shared their home with needy relatives and focused on day-to-day survival. When the United States entered World War II in 1941, the economy improved rapidly and the marriage rate increased dramatically. As more and more young men went off to war, the age of first-time brides and grooms dropped. After the war ended in 1945, the economy continued to grow and the age at which couples tied the knot continued to fall.

Since the mid-1950s, however, the median age at first marriage has been rising, with the biggest increases occurring since 1980. In 2008, the median age at first marriage was 27.6 years for men and 25.9 years for women. In 2008, 59 percent of men had not married by the time they reached their 30th birthdays, while 45.5 percent of women remained single at 30 years of age.

As F. Philip Rice, professor emeritus at the University of Maine-Orono, observes in *Intimate Relationships, Marriages, and Families,* people may be delaying marriage for several reasons, including increased opportunities for nonmarital sexual intercourse, increased acceptance of cohabitation, and less societal disapproval of single people. Rice suggests that many young adults are waiting to complete college and find their first job before marrying. In addition, women are now encouraged to develop identities outside of marriage and pursue careers and economic self-sufficiency both in and out of marriage.

However, most people do eventually marry. In 2008, according to Census Bureau data, only 19.7 percent of men and 13.5 percent of women had never married by the time they were 45 years old. The trend toward delayed marriage is significant because age at first marriage is the strongest predictor of marital success. Those who marry later are more likely to have a lasting marriage.

MARRIAGE AMONG WORKING COUPLES

In most marriages today, both spouses engage in paid work outside of the home. In the **dual-earner** family, both spouses are part of the labor force. According to the Census Bureau, in 1960, only 18 percent of women who had a child less than one year of age worked outside the home. By 2008, 46.2 percent of women with a child less than one year of age were in the labor force.

The dual-career family is a subset of the dual-earner family. While in most marriages today, both partners work outside the home, dual-career families are far less common. Both partners in these families are committed to both their professional and family lives. They constantly juggle roles and responsibilities. Pursuit of a career requires commitment and continuous professional development. For most professionals, having a career means full-time employment with little time away from the job and significant responsibilities on the job. The greater time commitment means they have less time to give to their mate and children.

Finding and paying for adequate child care is a challenge for many dual-earner families. In 2004, these parents paid on average more than $7,000 annually for child care, according to a study by Runzheimer International, a consulting firm. The cost of care in a caregiver's home, averaged $9,100 per year, while the annual cost of a live-in nanny was $27,664. The cost of day care varies by location and the child's age. As of 2007, the National Association of Child Care Resource and Referral Agencies (NACCRRA) listed the average annual day care costs as $8,150 for babies and toddlers and $6,423 for preschoolers. Although government-subsidized child-care programs offer services on a sliding scale basis, dual-earner couples may earn too much to qualify. In addition, many child-care facilities offer services only during standard working hours, which can pose problems for some working couples, especially those on night or evening shifts. Schedule limitations may also affect parents whose jobs require travel, those who work extra hours to complete projects, and those who are required to attend weekend seminars and continuing education courses.

Both dual-earner and dual-career couples balance the combined demands of marriage, child rearing, career, home, and friendships. Despite these challenges, there are tangible benefits to living in a two-income family. Most dual-earner couples enjoy higher incomes and a higher standard of living. In a study published in 2001 in the *Journal of Marriage and the Family,* sociologists Stacey J. Rogers and Danelle D. DeBoer found that as the income of women rises, so does their overall level of marital satisfaction and well-being.

In a 2003 study, also published in the *Journal of Marriage and the Family,* Rogers and her colleague Dee C. May found that job satisfaction and marital happiness were closely related. Rogers and May looked at data from 12 years of interviews with 2,034 married couples. As partners became happier in their marriages, they also became more satisfied with their jobs; when marital happiness decreased, so did job satisfaction at work. Marital happiness had a greater influence on job satisfaction than job satisfaction did on marital happiness. Both men and women were affected about equally. Rogers and May concluded that findings were consistent with previous research that showed the centrality of marital relationships in people's lives.

Q & A

Question: What can I do to reduce the chance that I will divorce?

Answer: Wait to marry, go to college, and delay having your first child until you've been married for at least seven months. According to data from the U.S. Census Bureau, almost half of all women who marry before the age of 18 divorce within 10 years, while less than a quarter of those who wait until they are 25 or older to marry divorce within the same time period. A second important predictor of divorce is education level. White men who have completed five or more years of college, and white women who have completed four years of college are the least likely to divorce. The timing of the birth of the first child in a family is another important predictor of divorce. Women who give birth within seven months of their marriage are twice as likely to divorce as those who wait to have their first child.

Many women who work report greater satisfaction with their lives overall, especially if they enjoy their job and their spouse is willing to help with household tasks and child care. In a study published in 2002 by the *Journal of Marriage and the Family,* a team of researchers led by sociologist Mary Maguire Klute found that the type of job a person holds influences marital equality, which in turn is an important predictor of overall happiness. Klute examined the relationship between the experiences of husbands and wives at work and their attitudes about and behaviors in marriage. She found that people who worked in jobs that required self-direction—for instance, making independent decisions, thinking for oneself, and setting one's own standards for behavior—were more likely to adopt more equal, or **egalitarian** arrangements in their marriages. These couples divided household tasks and child care more equally than did couples whose jobs required conformity—for instance, being neat, on time, and otherwise complying with standards set by authority figures. More egalitarian attitudes and behaviors in marriage, in turn, contributed to greater marital happiness.

MARRIAGE AMONG SAME-SEX COUPLES

In November 2003, the Supreme Judicial Court of Massachusetts ruled that the state could not refuse to allow gay and lesbian couples to marry. In response to an appeal, the court confirmed its decision that barring gays and lesbians from marriage was a violation of the state's constitution. The United States Supreme Court upheld the decision on May 17, 2004, and many same-sex couples rushed to the altar.

As of the end of 2009, the Defense of Marriage Acts are currently in place in the majority of states, defining marriage as the union between a man and a woman. Across the country, voters supported legislation to amend each state constitution that banned gay marriage. These amendments were in response to the 2003 Massachusetts overturning of the gay marriage ban due to the decision that it violated equal rights guarantees in the Massachusetts state constitution. Recently, however, a minority of states have amended their state constitution to support equal rights for same-sex couples. Some states extend to same-sex couples the same rights, protections, benefits, and obligations that heterosexual couples are afforded through marriage, and some other states have registration procedures for same-sex couples that grant them limited benefits. However, even the most extensive protections for gay and lesbian couples fall short of those afforded by legal marriages.

Marriage confers about 1,400 benefits, usually composed of about 400 state benefits and 1,000 federal benefits. These benefits include rights such as joint parenting, joint adoption, status of next-of-kin for hospital visits and medical decisions, dissolution and divorce protections for community property and child support, and benefits such as annuities, pension plans, Social Security, and Medicare.

The last half of the 20th century saw profound shifts in the structure and function of marriage and family life in the United States. Many unmarried couples are living together in domestic partnerships, often as a prelude to marriage. Men and women are waiting to marry until they are in their mid-to-late 20s. Several factors may contribute to delays in marriage, including increased opportunities for nonmarital sexual intercourse, increased acceptance of cohabitation, and less societal disapproval of single people. Among married couples, the two-income family has become increasingly common. Two-income couples often face challenges in managing their time and caring for children.

As more women enter the workforce, gender roles are being transformed within families. Women are sharing economic responsibilities, while men are taking on more household tasks and child care responsibilities. Same-sex couples are allowed to marry in Massachusetts and form civil unions or domestic partnerships in Vermont and California. However, gays and lesbians in most states are still fighting for the right to marry.

See also: Adoption; Day Care; Divorce and Families; Families, Blended; Families, Racially Mixed; Family, The New; Family, The Traditional; Gay Parents; Media and the Family; Single-Parent Families; Stepparents; Teenage Parents

FURTHER READING
Strong, Bryan. *The Marriage and Family Experience: Intimate Relationships in a Changing Society.* Florence, Ky.: Wadsworth Thompson Learning, 2010.

■ MEDIA AND THE FAMILY
The mass media includes radio, television, films, the Internet, books, newspapers, and magazines.

IMPACT ON CHILDREN
Messages sent to children in any form can be positive or harmful. The Kaiser Family Foundation reported in 2006 that children watch an average of 4,000 hours of television before they even enter kindergarten. In fact, they found that more than 40 percent of children under two years old watch television every day. Today, modern technology allows 24-hour access to the media. The Kaiser Foundation reported in a 2010 press release that research shows that children ages eight to 18 are spending more than 53 hours a week on entertainment media. That comes out to almost eight hours a day. Many experts believe the number is low, mainly because people are exposed to media messages not only through active viewing but also through passive exposure.

After a thorough review of the research, the American Academy of Pediatrics (AAP) argues that exposure to media has both benefits and risks. The benefits include increased access to information. For example, learning has been revolutionized as a result of access to the Internet. Social relationships both within the family and with friends often center on the shared experience of viewing popular programs or news events. Families today have greater understanding of global events and other cultures because of their access to news from around the world.

While experts recognize the educational and social benefits of exposure to media, they express greater concern over the risks of too much exposure. The research compiled by the AAP lists several downsides to increased exposure to media. More than a thousand studies show an increased risk of aggressive behavior in certain children and adolescents as a result of exposure to violent media messages. The AAP research review also found a connection between the time spent viewing TV programs, playing video games, or working on the computer and childhood obesity.

In 2007, the Kaiser Family Foundation released results from the largest study to date examining food advertising to kids. The research showed that children between the ages of eight and 18 are exposed to an average of 21 ads a day, or more than 7,600 ads a year. Of these ads, the foundation discovered that 34 percent of the food ads aimed at this age group are for candy and snacks, while 10 percent were for fast food. Although researchers examined more than 8,000 food ads marketed to this group, none was for fruits and vegetables.

Additionally, authors in a 2010 article in the journal *Pediatrics* explain that almost every concern that health professionals and parents have about teens, such as aggression, risky sexual behavior, drug and alcohol abuse, and eating disorders, can be affected by exposure to "old" media of television, movies, and magazines and also "new" media of Web sites and social networking, computer and video games, and cell phone applications.

FAMILY PROGRAMS ON TV

The nonprofit organization Center for Screen Time Awareness (CSTA) tries to raise awareness of the impact of television on family life. They recommend that parents decrease the amount of time that children spend watching television and promote alternatives such as family dinners or game nights.

The Nielsen Company measures media usage, and a 2009 report on teens found that their television viewing is up 6 percent, and they are spending an average of 11 hours each month online. The APA explains that if a child is watching television he or she is probably not engaged in any of the following: asking questions, solving problems, being creative, exercising initiative, practicing eye-hand coordination, practicing motor skills, thinking critically, logically, and analytically, practicing communication skills, or playing interactive games with other children or adults. The group recommends no television viewing for children under the age of two and no more than two hours per day of "high-quality" television programming for older children.

The Media Awareness Network points out that some television shows can benefit family life. Television programs that are educational and expose families to information about other cultures may help both children and their parents see the world from other points of view. News programs and documentaries may help students deepen or expand their understanding of subjects that they are studying in school. Watching television as a family, experts agree, allows parents to teach children to better understand the media messages they see and hear.

Q & A

Question: Can parents really do anything to minimize their children's exposure to negative media messages?

Answer: Yes, as Victor Strasburger reports in his 2010 article "Health Effects of Media on Children and Adolescents," experts say parents can do a lot to minimize the negative impact media messages have on children related to body image, substance use, sexuality, and violence. Limiting exposure to media messages, discussing media messages, and supervising the use of technology are important ways parents can influence exposure to media messages of all kinds.

ROLE MODELS AND FAMILIES

Media sources provide **role models** for children. Role models are people who are considered worthy of imitation. Role models can provide children with positive examples. However, some children choose individuals who set poor examples by abusing alcohol or drugs as their role models.

Many researchers are concerned that the media exposes children to poor role models. The Media Awareness Network is particularly troubled by the effects of role models in the fashion industry and the sexualized content often found in advertisements. Although the organization's research finds more positive role models for both boys and girls in the media than ever before, it remains concerned about the effects of negative role models on children's behavior. The organization continues to research the negative impact of unattainable and unrealistic beauty expectations for girls and young women. Studies have shown these images can attribute to poor body image and dissatisfaction as well as eating disorders in some girls.

Fact Or Fiction?

Children prefer to play video games and watch television over reading books for pleasure.

The Facts: While many children enjoy video games, the computer, and television, they are still engaged in reading. The Kaiser Family Foundation reported in 2010 that although the amount of time children spent with magazines or newspapers dropped between 1999 and 2009, the number of children reading magazines and newspapers online has increased. Also, the AAP reported that children who read more do better on verbal and math tests. In fact, researchers at the University of Michigan reported that each additional hour spent reading turned into half of a point higher on the child's test scores, and those half-points add up.

MEDIA LITERACY

The Center for Media Literacy is a nonprofit educational organization whose aim it is to educate people about the influence of media on families. The group's definition of media literacy or media education is widely used: "Media literacy is a 21st century approach to education. It provides a framework to access, analyze, evaluate and create messages in a variety of forms—from print to video to the Internet. Media literacy builds an understanding of the role of media in society as well as essential skills of inquiry and self-expression necessary for citizens of a democracy." Experts including the American Academy of Pediatrics (AAP) agree that the negative effects of media on children can be minimized and the positive effects maximized when parents engage in media education with children.

The Centers for Disease Control and Prevention, the Substance Abuse and Mental Health Services Administration (SAMHSA), the AAP, the National Education Association (NEA) Health Information Network, and the U.S. Department of Health and Human Services (HHS) all have studies showing that media education or media literacy may result in young people becoming less vulnerable to the negative aspects of media exposure. In the AAP review of research, experts state, "A media-educated person will be able to limit use of media; make positive media choices; select creative alternatives to media consumption; develop critical thinking and viewing skills; and understand the political, social, economic, and emotional implications of all forms of media."

See also: Communication Styles and Families; Family Rules; Violence and the Family

FURTHER READING
Durham, M. Gigi. *The Lolita Effect: The Media Sexualization of Young Girls and What We Can Do About it.* New York: Overlook TP, 2009.
Larson, Mary S. *Watch It!: What Parents Need to Know to Raise Media-Smart Kids.* Highland City, Fla.: Rainbow Books, 2009.
McCall, Jeffrey. *Viewer Discretion Advised: Taking Control of Mass Media Influences.* Lanham, Md.: Rowman & Littlefield, 2009.
Rideout, Vicky. *Zero to Six: Electronic Media in the Lives of Infants, Toddlers, and Preschoolers.* Menlo Park, Calif.: Kaiser Family Foundation, 2003.
Steyer, James P. *The Other Parent: The Inside Story of the Media's Effect on Our Children.* New York: Atria, 2003.
Strasburger, Victor C. *Children, Adolescents and Media.* New York: Sage Publications, 2002.
Winn, Marie. *The Plug-In Drug: Television, Computers and Family Life.* New York: Penguin, 2002.

■ PETS IN THE FAMILY

Pets are tame animals kept by a family as companions. Many families all over the world keep pets such as dogs, cats, birds, and fish. Some even own more exotic pets like monkeys, raccoons, alligators, and pythons. Some families regard such farm animals as horses, rabbits, and llamas as family pets as well.

Fact Or Fiction?

The domestic dogs that we keep as pets developed from the wolf.

The Facts: Although pet dogs did develop from wolves, dogs have changed as a result of thousands of years of involvement with humans. In the beginning, humans may have raised wolf cubs as guards. Through generations of human selection and random breeding, those wolves became domesticated, or tamed. North American wolves were ancestors to some dog breeds, such as the Alaskan Malamute, while Asian and European wolves were the stock for other breeds. DNA testing has traced these links.

For many Americans, it's impossible to picture a home without a dog or cat. Pets are great companions. The Humane Society of the United States gathered pet ownership data from their 2009–2010 National Pet Owners Survey. They found that there are 77.5 million pet dogs in America and almost 94 million pet cats. Two issues surrounding the decision to acquire a pet include allergies and the responsibility of taking care of the animal.

CHILDREN'S IMMUNE RESPONSE AND PETS

When a human comes into contact with an irritant, such as cat saliva or fur, the immune system in the body responds to it. The individual's reaction to the irritant is known as an **immune response** or immune reaction. If contact with a cat or dog results in watery eyes, a stuffy nose, asthma, or a skin rash, a person is said to have an allergic reaction to the animal.

A 2008 study published in the journal *Pediatric Allergy and Immunology* supports previous research that suggests that an early exposure to furry pets may decrease the chance of developing an allergy later in life. Previously, pediatricians believed that early exposure to cats and dogs would create more sensitivity as children got older. However, since the early 1990s, the opposite has been found to be true. The 2008 article supports the notion that contact with pets early in life actually may be a protective factor in the development of allergies later. Interestingly, the authors of this study also found that exposure to dogs had a much greater impact than exposure to cats.

Another possible issue in pet ownership is contact with an individual who suffers from asthma. Research published in 2008 in the journal *Allergy* explains that while early exposure to furry pets may prevent allergies from developing later on, particularly with dogs, this same exposure may increase the risk of asthma for young children in contact to dogs. While cat exposure may not protect children as much from allergies, that exposure has a lower chance of contributing to asthma problems later in life.

Owning a cat or a dog, therefore, can have both positive and negative effects on the allergy and immune systems of family members living with the pet. In fact, some studies indicate that not only children but also adults can benefit from having a pet, especially owning a dog. Dog owners also find social support and access to more walking and outdoor activities, which are beneficial to one's health.

TEACHING RESPONSIBILITY

Pets provide an opportunity to teach children responsibility. Children need to be shown just how dependent animals are on them for food, water, and exercise. People are not born knowing how to treat and care for pets, however. Children under 10 are rarely able to care for a cat or dog on their own. They may not realize how often a bird needs to eat to stay alive, that a turtle needs meat along with vegetable matter to survive, or that cats must have a bowl of water to drink.

Q & A ——————————————————————

Question: What is the ASPCA?

Answer: The American Society for the Prevention of Cruelty to Animals (ASPCA) tries to prevent cruelty to animals by offering national programs in humane education, through public awareness and government advocacy, and by offering shelter and medical services for and placement of unclaimed animals. The New York City headquarters includes a full-service animal hospital, behavior center, adoption facility, and humane law enforcement department.

Since 1866, the ASPCA has been committed to alleviating pain, fear, and suffering in all animals. It is the oldest humane organization in the United States and was founded by Henry Bergh, a philanthropist and diplomat who recognized the inhumane treatment suffered by many animals throughout the nation. The ASPCA is a privately funded, not-for-profit corporation.

A parent who understands how to care for pets can provide a good role model for his or her children. Parents and children can work together to keep their pet healthy.

If children become lax in caring for a pet, they should be reminded of their responsibility to their pets. If reminding does not help, parents may have to take over the responsibility or find a new home for the animal. In 2007, an article in the *International Journal of Artificial Intelligence in Education* pointed to the positive effects of pet ownership on children in all cultures, stating that people are naturally drawn to having a pet. The authors reported that children are especially fond of the idea of pets who can have a huge impact on a child's development in areas such as physiological health, psychological support, personality development, and social competence. However, pets should not suffer from lack of food or care because a child does not shoulder his or her responsibility.

The Humane Society of the United States warns against animal abuse. Intentional and repeated abuse of animals by older children should be viewed as a serious matter. A child who abuses is not just going through a phase. Studies show that children who deliberately abuse animals will often later abuse other children, property, and adults.

TEENS SPEAK

My Dog Is Precious to Me

I always have my dog Copper. I'm not lonely when I'm with him. He goes running with me. I practice homework with him because he listens. He understands words in Spanish now. I'm shy, but when he's with me, I can talk easily to other people.

Everyone in my family likes Copper. In the morning, he licks my sister awake. He's fun to watch and he herds us around. As soon as he hears the keys to the van jingle, he runs out and circles the van until we're all inside and then he jumps into his seat in the center of the middle seat.

Sometimes Copper is bad. He lets the rabbit out of the cage to watch it run. He is also hilarious. When we drive by the cows on the university campus farm, Copper closes his eyes, lifts his nose, and breathes in the smell of the animals. He's that way when we pass the zoo, too. He really likes that smell.

All of us (mom, dad, and four kids) care about our dog. When he escapes, we worry and run around the neighborhood looking for him. When he's sick, we worry and worry. When I saw the small kids across the street dragging their dogs and flinging them around, I asked my mother to go over and talk to them. And she did. Having Copper makes me worry about all animals. I wish everyone would.

Pet owners are responsible for their pet's behavior. Every year about 4.7 million dog bites occur in the United States, according to the Centers for Disease Control and Prevention (CDC). Of the 800,000 people who will need medical attention each year for a dog bite, half are children. Dog bites are most common in children between the ages of five and nine and are more serious among young children. Probably because of their small size, they receive bites mainly on the head and neck. Teens and adults receive bites mainly on their hands and arms. The CDC suggests that a person not pet or make eye contact with an unfamiliar dog and not pet any dog without allowing it to see and sniff you first. Children and adults also need to learn how to approach a dog. When a strange dog comes near, they should remain quiet and calm. If they run or panic, the dog may run after them.

COMPANIONSHIP

Many people report feeling happier caring for a pet. Quite a bit of research has been conducted on the health benefits of pet ownership, so much so that researcher Javier Virues-Ortega looked at all of the research in 2006 and found that while some contradictions do exist, two major theories seem to hold true. He discovered that based on all of the previous research, there is evidence to show lower cardiovascular levels, such as blood pressure, in pet owners. He also confirmed that having a pet can help lower stress levels and help the owner to respond to new stressors in a more productive manner.

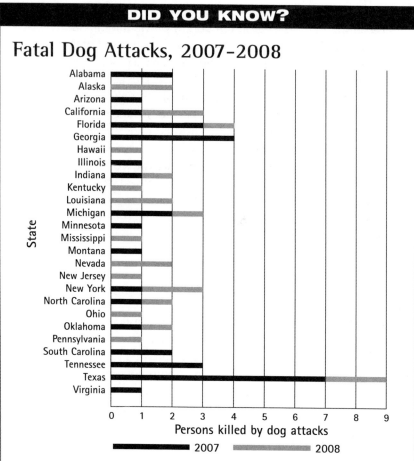

DID YOU KNOW?

Fatal Dog Attacks, 2007–2008

Owning a pet comes with the responsibility of controlling a pet's behavior in order to avoid injuries to both pets and people. Some dog attacks also result in fatalities, and those numbers have been rising. In the United States in the 1980s and 1990s, the average was 17 fatal attacks each year. However, there were 33 deaths in 2007, 23 deaths in 2008, and 30 in 2009.

Source: Dogbitelaw.com, 2009.

Pets provide more than companionship. Dogs and even rabbits visit hospitals and nursing facilities to provide patients and elderly residents with attention. Specially trained dogs assist people with disabilities, helping them handle everyday tasks. Seeing-eye dogs guide those who are blind. Other dogs hear for their human companions.

Still others help by picking up items from the ground or alerting their companion to a possible seizure.

Some libraries are implementing a new program called R.E.A.D., which stands for Reading Education Assistance Dogs. The nonprofit group Intermountain Therapy Animals started the program in 1999, and now it exists in the United Kingdom, Canada, and across the United States. It allows children to improve both their communication and reading skills by reading out loud to registered therapy dogs.

Pets can provide companionship and support for their owners. The only drawbacks are allergies and the need for owners to assume responsibility for their pets.

See also: Adoption; Death in the Family; Family Rules; Family Traditions

FURTHER READING

Gerstenfeld, Sheldon. *ASPCA: A Complete Guide to Dogs.* San Francisco: Chronicle Books, 1999.

Herriot, James. *All Creatures Great and Small.* New York: St. Martin's Press, 1972.

Humane Society of the United States. *Complete Guide to Cat Care.* New York: St. Martin's Press, 2002.

Puotinen, C. J. *Encyclopedia of Natural Pet Care,* rev. ed. Los Angeles: Keats Publishing, 1998.

■ PUBERTY AND SEXUAL DEVELOPMENT

The process by which a male or female child enters sexual maturity and becomes capable of reproduction. The onset of puberty brings about different physical changes in the two genders, new **sexual phenomena** that both boys and girls experience, as well as various emotional changes. Puberty arrives at a time of life known as **adolescence**, which is the period of transition from childhood to adulthood.

Contrary to what some people think, puberty is not something that happens all at once, like a switch being thrown. It is a process that takes a different amount of time for every person but almost always takes years from start to finish. Similarly, there is no one "normal" age for puberty to begin or end: The range is wide, and it is quite different for boys and girls.

The nature of puberty is such that its variations can cause stress for boys and girls who mature early or late. That just adds to the stress inherent, or natural, in a young body that is evolving into an adult body, complete with adult **hormones,** drives, desires, and emotions. As a result, puberty can be a difficult time, especially for those who lack basic information and therefore are needlessly frightened or frustrated by the physical and emotional changes their bodies are undergoing.

ONSET OF PUBERTY

Sexual maturation is a personal matter, and every person is different. However, research indicates that puberty typically starts between ages eight and 13 in girls and ages 10 and 15 in boys. The differences in onset can lead to great discomfort among groups of boys and girls who, to that point, have essentially been at the same level of maturity for years.

An amazing array of factors determines when puberty begins. Researchers have learned that, in addition to a person's **genes,** which obviously play a key role, factors such as what you eat and how active you are can help determine when puberty begins. Even stress at home or at school or the size of your family can be factors in starting the process. The important idea to remember is that nobody gets to choose when puberty begins, nor is there anything a person can do to rush it or slow its onset.

There is another argument against the idea of "normal" when it comes to puberty. As with any group, there will be boys and girls who reach puberty earlier than everyone else, and there will be those who do not begin to develop sexually until later than their friends. There is nothing abnormal about the differences; they simply represent the range of individual experiences. With rare exceptions, the ultimate result is that, by about age 17 for girls and age 19 for boys, everyone has completed the process and is an adult, biologically speaking.

PHYSICAL CHANGES

Puberty starts when the body begins secreting hormones, which are the chemicals designed to bring about the changes in the body which lead to sexual maturity. Some of the changes are similar in both boys and girls, but because their bodies are so different, and there are different hormones involved, there are also specific changes that affect each of the two genders.

For girls, who usually enter puberty at a younger age than boys, the changes are often unwelcome, inconvenient, and even a little frightening. Some of the changes are obvious to everyone: a girl's

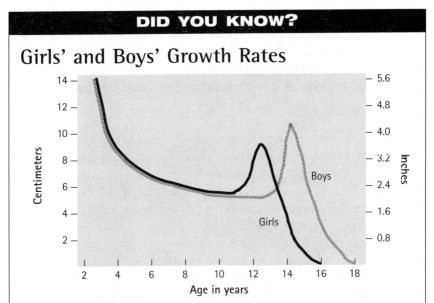

DID YOU KNOW?

Girls' and Boys' Growth Rates

During puberty, both boys and girls experience growth spurts—but, as this chart shows, the phenomenon tends to occur about two years earlier for girls.

Source: Centers for Disease Control and Prevention, via Short Persons Support, at http://www.shortsupport.org/Health/Children/spurt.gif.

breasts begin to develop and grow larger; her hips often widen; the waist narrows; and many girls will experience a growth spurt that sends them soaring over boys of comparable age.

There are other changes as well. Everyone has hair on their bodies, even as children, but most girls will start to see more, and often darker, hair, on their arms, legs, under their arms, and in their "bikini area," or the **mons veneris**, the external fatty tissue that protects the pubic bone. Many girls notice that their hair and skin more easily become oily. Acne is often a problem as well, and sweat might become a problem for the first time, requiring the use of deodorant.

Q & A

Question: Does everyone get pimples during puberty?

Answer: According to the Centers for Disease Control and Prevention, about 85 to 90 percent of all boys and girls have acne during puberty. The hormones that bring about sexual development cause the oil glands to become more active, and that causes acne or pimples on the face, upper back, and upper chest. It's not a matter of being dirty—almost everyone deals with the same problem. The pimples start around the beginning of puberty and continue for a few years, but they usually go away in time.

Most significant is when **menstruation** begins, the monthly shedding of the lining of the **uterus**. Typically, on a 28-day menstrual cycle, a girl will begin to be **fertile** for a portion of the time; about five days of the cycle will involve her "period," which is a regeneration of sorts. When menstruation begins, a woman is sexually mature and is capable of conceiving a child.

For boys, many of the signs and characteristics of puberty are the same as for girls: Body hair, for example, will appear; acne may become a problem, along with oil on the skin and sweating; and growth spurts will be common. Boys, however, are more likely to see growth in a wider variety of body parts, including hands, feet, and even ears. Unlike a girl, a boy's hips will narrow and his shoulders will widen; these changes might be subtle or extreme, depending on the boy. Two other experiences unique to boys are a change in voice, usually to a deeper voice, and the appearance of facial hair.

A boy also will notice growth in his **penis** and the development of **testes**, which actually descend to the **scrotum** from within the body. Soon thereafter, a boy has reached sexual maturity and has the capability of fathering a child.

SEXUAL PHENOMENA

Although the arrival of puberty can be an intimidating and confusing time for both genders, boys have a few issues of their own. Boys will begin to experience **erections**. An erection occurs when a boy is thinking sexual thoughts or feeling sexual desire, but often it will occur for no reason at all. This can be embarrassing, but it is completely normal and is something that generally will pass as puberty ends.

Most boys also will have nocturnal emissions, also known as "wet dreams." This is an **ejaculation** during sleep, with or without a sexual dream accompanying it. It is a perfectly normal occurrence; some boys experience it once, some several times. Although a bit inconvenient, uncomfortable, and embarrassing, it is harmless and something that generally passes with the completion of puberty.

TEENS SPEAK

Am I out of Control?

I'm an only child, and I just turned 11; I pay attention in health class, so I guess what's happening to me is called puberty. I notice some changes in my body, and I've seen other boys in the locker room after gym class, so I think I know what to expect. But what confuses me more is the way I feel.

I have a lot of girls who are friends, but I'm starting to have feelings about some of them that I can't quite understand. I get nervous around them, which I never did before. I don't know too much about sex, since my parents are very religious, but I can't stop thinking about certain girls. I'm getting yelled at in class because I daydream all the time, and a lot of the time I'm thinking about them.

I have never had a temper before, but I notice I'm getting in trouble for talking back to my parents. I get angry so much easier than I used to. I don't really know why most of the time—sometimes I wonder if I'm out of control.

I talked to my friend Dean, who is 13, and he said he felt the same way and even got into fights on the way to school for a while, but then he just lost interest in fighting. I wonder if that will happen to me, if my temper will get me into fights with classmates. I don't want to fight, but I wonder if I will anyway.

I wish I had an older brother to talk to about this. I would feel funny asking my dad or anyone at school. But I can't stop worrying that things will get worse. Am I ever going to feel in control again?

For girls, most of the sexual phenomena involve menstruation and its related symptoms. Cramps are most significant; they are caused by the increased production of hormones during the girl's period, and that causes the muscles of the uterus to contract. Other problems can include back pain, bloating, nausea, diarrhea, or fatigue.

Some girls also experience **premenstrual syndrome**, or PMS, just before their periods. The symptoms of PMS include irritability, difficulty in sleeping, bloating, anxiety, and odd cravings. Once a girl's period starts for the month, these symptoms often lessen or disappear.

EMOTIONAL CHANGES

While dealing with the fallout of puberty, there is an added issue: emotions, fueled by hormones, can run amok in both boys and girls. Both genders can become more self-conscious, more prone to feeling emotions much more deeply (and acting out on those emotions more readily), and confused about the changes taking place and where they lead.

Again, this is a normal part of puberty. It may be difficult, in the midst of these changes, to accept that things will change one day, but they will. Adult emotions are something new, and most adolescents will grow into them, just as they grow into their adult bodies.

Puberty is also a time when sexual identity begins to come into focus. Some experimentation is normal and does not necessarily predict a person's sexual orientation. Sexual desire, a new feeling, can become overwhelming at times for either gender. It is important to remember that these feelings are not unusual. It is always a good idea to find someone you trust to discuss them with: a doctor, a counselor, a family member, or another responsible adult. Sometimes older siblings of the same gender can talk you through the difficulties of puberty, because they went through it themselves—and survived.

See also: Independence

FURTHER READING

Harris, Robie H. *It's Perfectly Normal: Changing Bodies, Growing Up, Sex, and Sexual Health.* Cambridge, Mass.: Candlewick Press, 1996.

Madaras, Lynda, and Area Madaras. *The "What's Happening to My Body?" Book for Girls.* New York: Newmarket Press, 2007.

Madaras, Lynda, Area Madaras, and Dane Saavidra. *The "What's Happening to My Body?" Book for Boys.* New York: Newmarket Press, 2007.

■ RELIGION AND THE FAMILY

Religion is a formal expression of or institution based on a belief in a divine or higher power that controls human destiny. In 2000, Harris Interactive, a national polling service, found that 94 percent of

Americans claim that they believe in God. According to the Institute for Youth Development, religious faith is also strong among young people. Their studies show that 94 percent of teens say they believe in God and nearly nine in 10 teens consider their religious beliefs important to them.

According to the researcher Ellen Idler from Rutgers University, spirituality and religion have positive impacts on a person's health and well-being that span one's entire life. She finds that practicing spiritual and religious beliefs can make a person healthier both physically and emotionally.

Also, in a study in 2006, Dr. Daniel Hall reported that regular religious attendance can have a very significant effect on one's physical health. Hall compared the estimated added life years attributed to weekly religious ceremony attendance, regular physical activity, and taking blood pressure medicine. The results showed that weekly religious services could account for two to three more years of life, regular physical exercise could provide an additional three to five years of life; and blood pressure–reducing medication could give two and a half to three and a half more years. Dr. Hall then looked at the average costs of these life-extending interventions for each year that they added and found regular exercise to be the cheapest extender, at $2,000 to $6,000, followed by religious exercise at $3,000 to $10,000. The use of blood pressure medication accounted for approximately $4,000 to $14,000 for each year added to life.

REARING CHILDREN IN FAITH

In many families, religion is an important part of family life. Their faith helps parents manage both work and family and is a vital resource in teaching their children about faith and morality. Religion can also strengthen family relationships. Penny Edgell, professor of American religion and sociology at the University of Minnesota, found that despite ongoing social change, religion and families still go hand and hand.

Raising children with faith or in a faith community is important to many families. In other families, religion may be a source of tension. Debates over religion within the family have been going on for generations and continue today. Whether a person focuses on organized religion or a sense of spirituality and faith, beliefs are individual and personal.

In 2009, the Barna Research Group, a marketing research firm serving nonprofit organizations and various media and financial corporations, found that of the 1,000 adults polled in their survey, 80 percent remembered regularly attending Sunday School or another religious training institution before the age of 12. Religious education is defined as a tool used to transmit knowledge and values pertaining to a particular faith. Exposure to the stories, beliefs, theologies, and practices of a family's religion will give children the tools they need to make up their own minds about life's big questions.

The National Study of Youth and Religion (NSYR) is an ongoing project whose purpose is to research the influence of religion and spirituality on the lives of adolescents in the United States. Their findings suggest that religiously involved families are more likely to have stronger relationships than families that are not religiously active.

According to Mark Baker, clinical director of the LaVie Counseling Center, children benefit from learning that there is something greater than themselves in the spectrum of life. The Barna Research Group conducted additional research in 2009 and found that almost 90 percent of the respondents viewed their religious faith as very or somewhat important in their lives. Almost 75 percent reported that their faith was becoming more important.

However, not all parents raise their children with a similar devotion to religion. A 2007 study done by the same organization found that among the parents who considered themselves Christian in the survey, only 14 percent reported their "spiritual challenge" was to raise their children with a strong faith. Thirty percent of these parents said that helping their children to become more spiritual was very daunting.

Parents interested in teaching religion, faith, or spirituality should begin by sharing their own beliefs. Conversations are meaningful when parents talk openly and honestly about faith and the mysteries of life. Every family is different when it comes to spiritual beliefs, so how parents proceed with religious teaching is personal. Laying a strong foundation for ongoing communication is an important step in this process of introducing religion.

Q & A

Question: Should parents teach their children their own beliefs or wait until their children are old enough to make their own decision about religion?

Answer: In 2007, an international conference on religion that was reviewed by the journal *Religious Studies Review* declared that there are physiological and social practicalities for the need of religious education for children but that there must be a happy medium and a child should have a choice. While many parents oversee the spiritual direction of their children in churches and synagogues, others struggle on their own. Parents are looking for a way to teach religion that gives children the best of what religion has to offer but does not build resentment.

INTERFAITH FAMILIES

While statistics are elusive on the exact number of interfaith families in the United States, many faith communities believe that the number is rising, particularly among young adults. Some research, like that of Kate McCarthy, states that more than 20 percent of Americans marry outside of their faith. McCarthy also finds that certain religions seem to be more tolerant and open to this action than others. The United Jewish Communities organization cites that, according to previous National Jewish Population Surveys, the rate for interfaith marriages between Jewish and non-Jewish individuals has been increasing. For those who married before 1970, the rate for Jewish out-of-faith marriage was 13 percent, but around 1970, the number rose to 28 percent. Then, by the early 1980s, the rate had increased to almost 40 percent, and by the mid-90s, the rate of interfaith marriages in the Jewish community was almost 50 percent.

According to Interfaith Family, an online community, interfaith families should speak openly about how to mix and mesh traditions such as weddings, ceremonies, and holiday celebrations as well as how to raise children. For many interfaith families, the religious goal is to honor the distinctiveness of each religious tradition and not to try and create a new blend.

Interfaith marriages pose challenges for families, religious establishments, faith communities, and society at large. Often, families feel lonely and isolated from faith communities and sometimes from extended families, too.

Fact Or Fiction?

Growing up in an interfaith family is too confusing to children.

The Facts: When parents take an active role in teaching children about their family's faith, children need not be confused. Robin Margolis, an interfaith religious educator and director of the Half-Jewish Network, says that the best way to make growing up in an interfaith family a positive experience is to give children information about both religions. She recommends that instead of blending religious beliefs, expose children to the rich traditions of both. Later, she says it is important for parents to respect their adult children's choice regarding religion.

Holidays and faith-based celebrations can present what is referred to in many interfaith families as the "December Dilemma." Mary Rosenbaum, from the Kentucky-based interfaith family resource called the Dovetail Institute, explains that holidays require negotiation. Not only are there competing faith-based traditions, but many times each parent will have familial traditions that differ from the other. Rosenbaum explains that it is important to have holiday discussions before children are born and even to consider how those decisions will affect the extended family members.

See also: Death in the Family; Family Traditions; Gay Parents

FURTHER READING
Gruzen, Lee F. *Raising Your Jewish/Christian Child: How Interfaith Parents Can Give Children the Best of Both of Their Heritages.* New York: Newmarket Press, 2001.
Schaper, Donna E. *Raising Interfaith Children: Spiritual Orphans or Spiritual Heirs.* New York: Crossroad Publishing, 1999.
Yust, Karen M. *Real Children, Real Faith.* New York: Jossey-Bass, 2004.

■ SINGLE-PARENT FAMILIES
A single-parent family is composed of a parent and one or more children. The parent may have never been married or have been widowed or divorced. Single-parent families face a number of financial, psychological, and societal challenges.

FINANCIAL ISSUES
According to the Census Bureau, 27 percent of all children in the United States are living in single-parent households. In 2008, the

nation was home to more than 11.6 million single parents. Of single-parent households, 84 percent are headed by a female, while males head about 16 percent. These households include a disproportionate number of African Americans. Sixty-four percent of African-American children under the age of 18 live with one parent or neither parent. In comparison, about 26 percent of white children under the age of 18 live with a single parent or neither parent.

Single parents face a host of challenges in raising their children. They must constantly balance the demands of their job, child care, and their own needs. All too often, they face financial difficulties. While both women and men who become single as a result of divorce or the death of a spouse often experience a drastic decrease in income, this decrease is often more significant for women. Census data reveals that in 2008, the average income of single-mother families was $39,660, while single-father families had an annual average income of $56,808. By comparison, two-parent families earned an average of $91,452 a year. In addition, the incomes of divorced women who receive full child support from their ex-partners are on average 25 percent lower than those of divorced men who receive child support payments.

Fact Or Fiction?

Marriage would solve single mothers' poverty problems.

The Facts: Researchers and policy makers agree that married women are less likely to be poor—in 2002, families with single mothers and their children made up half of all families in poverty—but they disagree about solutions to the problem. Programs that promote marriage for poor women are often touted as a way to help single women and their children leave welfare rolls. However researchers at the Institute for Women's Policy Research (IWPR) have found that single mothers are poorer for three primary reasons: they are likely to be paid less than men for the same work, to work at lower-paying jobs, and to work fewer hours than men because they assume more responsibilities for child care. IWPR researchers maintain that equal pay for women and men, more education, and child-care subsidies are the keys to helping single mothers move out of poverty.

Single parents are more likely to be poor than married couples. The association between single parenthood and poverty is demonstrated strikingly in the District of Columbia, where two out of every three children do not live with married parents. Washington, D.C., also has one of the highest percentages of children living in poverty in the nation. Census Bureau data show that in 2002, 33 percent of children in Washington, D.C., lived below the federal poverty level of $14,494 for a family of three.

The Census Bureau reports that in 2009, 9.6 percent of all families in the nation lived in poverty. Of these families, 14.2 percent were married-couple families, 22.8 percent were male-headed single families, and 38.6 percent were female-headed. Children in these families were five times as likely to be living in poverty as those who lived with two parents. Families headed by a single male parent were less likely to be poor but still more likely to be in poverty than households headed by two adults. Of households headed by a single male, 525,000 were in poverty, representing 28.5 percent of all single-father families.

One reason that many single-parent families have less income than two-parent families may be that single parents are unable to work as many hours as married couples. Census Bureau data shows that between 1993 and 2001, the percentage of custodial parents employed in a full-time year-round job grew from 45.6 percent to 55.3 percent. In 2008, about 19 percent of custodial parents worked part-time or for part of the year. Custodial mothers were more likely than fathers to work part-time, although their full-time year-round employment increased to 53.2 percent. In contrast, 82 percent of custodial fathers were employed in full-time, year-round jobs in 2008.

Single mothers of all ethnic backgrounds and education levels face a formidable wage gap. In 2008, according to the Bureau of Labor Statistics, women who were employed full-time earned 80 cents for every dollar that men earned in similar jobs. Researchers from the Institute for Women's Policy Research (IWPR) predict that women will not earn the same pay for performing the same work, or **economic parity,** until 2050.

The discrepancy in wages is slightly greater for single parents. According to IWPR, working single mothers earn 71 percent of the hourly wages of working single fathers—even when both groups have similar levels of education. In analyzing census data, IWPR researchers found that single fathers tended to work in industrial, manufacturing, construction, and managerial jobs. In contrast, women tended to work in service jobs in restaurants, department stores, and hospitals.

The difference in jobs and wages leads to what researchers call "sex segregation" in the labor market. That segregation translates into a $5,000-a-year gap between low-income men and women.

IWPR researchers suggest that the need for child care, transportation, and special job skills may also affect a single parent's ability to find and keep a job that pays enough to maintain a household. Single parents who lack job skills and/or experience may need to enroll in a training program or attend college. They may also need to develop emotional and other support systems that will help them become effective heads of households and wage earners. Inadequate child care is often a barrier to a woman's full-time employment. To make ends meet, many single parents rely on a combination of wages, government assistance programs, and contributions from family and friends.

PSYCHOLOGICAL IMPACT

Like any other family, a single-parent family can provide a healthy environment for its members. Children thrive in a warm, supportive home, regardless of whether it is headed by one or two parents. Studies also suggest that children adjust better when they have a good relationship with a single parent than when they live with two parents who are in constant conflict. Parents who are inaccessible, rejecting, or hostile can be more damaging to children than absent parents.

However, many single-parent families face particular emotional and psychological challenges. In "The Diversity, Strength, and Challenges of Single-Parent Households," a 2003 review of recent research concerning single-parent families, psychologist Carol Anderson points to a large body of research on the most common challenges for single parents and their children. Those challenges include the need to "go it alone," cope with the loss of a relationship, and endure financial hardship—all of which leave single parents more vulnerable to psychological problems such as depression.

According to Anderson, several studies suggest that teens in single-parent families are more likely to drop out of high school and become a parent. As adults, they are more likely to be unemployed and rely on public assistance. However, as Anderson observes, many of these studies do not take into account other factors—including poverty (both before and after a parental divorce), moving to a new (and usually poorer and less safe) neighborhood, family size, ethnicity, and the single parent's educational level—all of which can affect a child's adjustment and well-being.

In 1994, sociologists Sara McLanahan and Gary Sandefur published the results of a study designed to examine the factors that may be responsible for children of single parents faring less well than those in two-parent families. Their analysis, published in *Growing Up with a Single Parent: What Hurts, What Helps,* showed that even after adjusting for differences in race, parent's education, family size, and neighborhood, children in single-parent families had more social, behavioral, and emotional problems than those living with two biological parents. The research showed little difference between single-parent families created by divorce and those that were the result of out-of-wedlock births.

McLanahan and Sandefur did find one important variable: family income. Their analysis showed that the loss in income that occurred when the custodial parent became a single parent—whether by divorce, death, or nonmarital birth—was the single most important factor for the decline in well-being of children in one-parent families. About half of the decline in children in single-parent families was due to a lower income.

Other studies have demonstrated that children in single-parent families are less likely to do well in school. McLanahan and Sandefur, for instance, found that children of single parents were 50 percent more likely to drop out of school than children in two-parent families. However, a study published in the *Journal of Educational Research* in 2004 suggests that children's performance in school seems to be more strongly affected by a parent's involvement, education, and abilities than his or her marital status.

Researchers led by Henry Ricciuti, professor of human development at Cornell University, assessed the school performances and behavior of 1,500 children of single mothers from white, black, and Hispanic families. The children were interviewed when they were six and seven years old and again when they were 12 and 13. In both sets of interviews, researchers found that living with a single mother did not affect a child's readiness for school or contribute to social or behavioral problems.

Researchers at Cornell also found that children's educational performance and behavior was most strongly affected by the mother's education and ability level. Less influential but still important were family income and the quality of the home environment. Those links were consistent across ethnic and racial groups. The researchers concluded that when single mothers are educated, have adequate income, expect positive achievement from their children, and have a network of social resources, single parenthood does not increase a child's risk of poor educational performance or behavior problems. However, the children of single mothers who lack those resources may indeed be at risk of poor academic performance, substance abuse, and delinquency.

In comparison to married parents, single parents have little relief from the responsibilities of parenting. In two-parent families, spouses typically rely on each other for social and emotional support. Spouses help each other with child care, transportation, and negotiating conflicting or competing demands. But most single parents, as Anderson observes, cope with child care, household responsibilities, work, and social life without the help of a partner. In 2008, a review in the *Journal of Divorce and Remarriage* examined studies that assessed the differences in the psychological well-being between intact and nonintact families. Findings showed that psychological well-being decreased in nonintact families relative to intact families.

TEENS SPEAK

I Live With a Single Dad

I've lived with my dad since my parents divorced about 10 years ago. I was six years old when they split up, and I remember feeling sad and confused for a long time afterwards. I didn't understand why my mom left, but I did know that they fought a lot before the divorce. My mom moved to an apartment and my dad and I stayed in our old house. I saw her on weekends and during holidays for the first year after they divorced. Then the consulting firm my mom works for transferred her to their office in France. My dad and I stayed in Phoenix, where he's a partner in a law firm. Dad and I get along pretty well. He's a great cook, and he's taught me how to cook Thai, Mexican, and a few other cuisines. We often have fun making a mess in the kitchen; sometimes we even clean it up. Both of us are lousy housekeepers, which is just as well. He has to travel out of town occasionally, so I sometimes stay with my friend Julia and her mom. But most of the time, he's around. He takes me to soccer practices and flute lessons, and he shows up at every one of my flute recitals. He does the best job he can at being both "mom" and "dad."

Sometimes though, I wish my mom were still around. Some things are hard to talk to my dad about. The hardest thing is explaining to my friends that I live with my dad and not my mom. About half of my friends' parents are divorced, and most of them live with their moms. Some of them also have stepfathers.

I spend a month each summer overseas with my mom and Jacques, the man she married about a year ago. Jacques has a daughter about my age, so my visits to France are fun and filled with lots of interesting things to do, and my mom will always be my mom. But my home is in Arizona with my dad.

Not surprisingly, considerable data show that single parents are more likely to experience loneliness. Sociologists suggest that there are two types of loneliness. People who experience **social isolation** feel lonely because they lack a social network of friends and acquaintances. Those who experience **emotional isolation** are lonely because they lack a single intense relationship.

Divorced, separated, and widowed people are more likely to experience both types of loneliness. In a 1991 study published in *Psychological Reports,* psychologists Randy Page and Galen Cole found that among adults who said they were lonely, 20 percent were divorced, 30 percent were separated, and 20 percent were widowed. Only 14.5 percent of the never-married said they felt lonely. Of married people, 4.6 percent reported feelings of loneliness. In an international survey published in the journal *Sociology* in 1998, Steven Stack, a sociologist at Wayne State University in Detroit, assessed the relationship between marital status and loneliness. Stack found similar patterns in 17 industrialized nations: the married were least lonely, and the divorced, separated, or widowed were the most lonely.

According to a 2008 study published in the *Journal of Family Issues,* loneliness in the single parent is less common in families whose family networks have a higher frequency of contact with close kin. Factors such as larger family network size and closer geographical proximity to other family members were found to be helpful in reducing the level of loneliness experienced by the single parent.

SOCIETAL VIEWS

With more than half of all marriages ending in divorce and an increasing number of unmarried women choosing to have children, the shame or disgrace once attached to single-parent families is lessening. More than 60 percent of children will live in a single-parent home before they reach the age of 18.

The changes in attitudes regarding single parents are reflected most strongly in the increasing number of unmarried women who choose to have children. Between 1940 and 1990, births to unmarried mothers in the United States increased from less than 4 percent to 28 percent. Between 1990 and 2007, the percentage of births to unmarried mothers rose from 28 to 39.7 percent, according to data from the National Center for Health Statistics. The most notable increases were among educated white women in professional positions. Among never-married, college-educated women, the birthrate doubled; among never-married women who work in a professional or managerial capacity, the birthrate tripled.

Many single mothers express concern about their marital status and how it affects their ability to cope as a mother. However, for some of these women, the desire to have a child outweighs the social, emotional, and financial challenges of single parenting.

GOVERNMENT ASSISTANCE

For many parents, the transition to single parenting means a loss of income, increased responsibilities, and a lack of job opportunities. Many single parents turn to the government for assistance for basic needs, child care, and health insurance. Government assistance programs can be divided into two general categories: those in which benefits are based on income level and need, and those in which benefits are based on work history, such as unemployment insurance or social security. Single parents can access these programs by contacting the local office of their state's human services or labor and employment departments.

Income level and need are used to determine whether a family qualifies for the following programs:

- Temporary Aid to Needy Families (TANF). In 1996, Congress passed the Personal Responsibility and Work Opportunity Reconciliation Act (PRWORA). Better known as welfare reform, the act was designed to reduce dependence on government benefits and increase paid employment and marriage. PRWORA replaced Aid for Families with Dependent Children (AFDC) program with TANF. Under AFDC, low-income single mothers were entitled to receive monthly payments as long as they had a child in their care. Under TANF, a person can receive cash assistance for no more than five years during his or her lifetime. Cash benefits vary depending on the state in which the person lives, but 99 percent of TANF recipients received a monthly payment of $351 or less in 2003. People who receive TANF benefits are also required to work, volunteer, or attend a vocational training program for at least 30 hours per week.

- Food stamps. Some single-parent families are eligible for food stamps, a program run by the U.S. Department of Agriculture (USDA). Families receive monthly assistance in buying food. The amount they receive is based on income and family size. Families do not receive cash. Instead they receive paper coupons or an electronic benefits transfer (EBT) card. Those who use an EBT card have an account established in their family's name. Every month, the government deposits money into that account to use when paying for groceries.

- Housing assistance. Housing assistance is available to low-income families through the Department of Housing and Urban Development (HUD). Eligibility is determined by the family's income and the median family income in the area in which they live. HUD defines low-income families as those whose income is less than 80 percent of the median income in the area. HUD offers several programs to these families, ranging from housing facilities and assistance in paying rent to home-buying and home renovations.

■ Child care. Low-income single-parent families may also be eligible for assistance with child-care. Eligible families can take advantage of subsidized child care services, usually through a certificate or a contract with a child care provider. The provider must meet basic health and safety requirements. Children three to five years old can enroll in Head Start, a national program that provides day care, education, and developmental services for low-income children and social services to their families. Each Head Start program is run by a community-based nonprofit organization or a school system. Intellectual, social, and emotional growth is promoted through a variety of learning experiences.

■ Health insurance. Low-income families may qualify for Medicaid and the state-run Children's Health Insurance Program (CHIP). Medicaid is a program run by both federal and state governments that provides health care to low-income people. Qualification requirements for Medicaid programs vary, but families must be below the federal poverty level, which is updated yearly and varies according to family size. The CHIP program was reauthorized when the president signed into law the Children's Health Insurance Program Reauthorization Act of 2009. CHIPRA finances CHIP through 2013. CHIPRA will preserve health care coverage for the millions of children who rely on CHIP today and provide the resources for states to reach millions of additional uninsured children. This legislation will help ensure the health and well-being of the nation's children. Qualification for assistance is defined by a family of four making less than $41,300 per year and who was without health insurance for six months before being enrolled. Children in families with slightly higher incomes may be covered under CHIP, which is designed to ensure that children at all income levels have access to health care. While the income limits in CHIP vary by state, in most states, they are set at about 200 percent of the poverty level.

Q & A

Question: Should I drop out of high school and go to work to help my single mom make ends meet?

Answer: Dropping out of high school to go to work may provide a short-term fix to your family's financial problems, but in the long run, it's not likely to help you and your family permanently move out of poverty. In fact, dropping out makes it more likely that you will find yourself struggling to make ends meet as you grow older. You are more likely to be able to help your mom and siblings in a substantial way if you finish high school and seek financial assistance to go to college. In the meantime, you and your family can investigate other options to make ends meet, including part-time work and government assistance programs designed for families like yours.

FAMILY SUPPORT

Many single parents depend on their extended families for emotional, physical, and financial support. About half of all low-income single mothers live with other adults, including their own parents, siblings, boyfriends, or roommates. Women who work full time are most likely to live with other adults of their own generation, while younger women are more likely to live with parents or grandparents.

In 2008, according to the Census Bureau, 6.6 million children were living with a grandparent. Six percent of white non-Hispanic children, 10 percent of Hispanic children, 14 percent of Asian children, and 14 percent of African-American children lived with a grandparent.

Single parents may be able to parent more effectively if they have the support of their extended families. In a study published in 2002 in the journal *Demography,* Thomas DeLeire and Ariel Kalil of the School of Public Policy Studies at the University of Chicago reported that teens may benefit from living in three-generation households. DeLeire and Kalil examined data from 11,213 teens who participated in the National Educational Longitudinal Survey. First, they determined what type of family the teen lived in when he or she was in eighth grade: married-parent, single-parent, extended family, and other possible structures (including two unmarried biological parents). Then they examined how well the teens were doing during their senior year in high school or two years after high school. The researchers looked for such indicators of well-being as substance abuse, sexual activity, high school graduation, and college attendance.

When they compared the teens' behaviors with the structures of their families, DeLeire and Kalil found that teens who lived in single-parent families were generally less likely to graduate from high school or attend college, more likely to smoke or drink, and more likely to begin sexual activity at an early age. However, teens who lived with a single parent and a grandparent showed developmental outcomes that were as good—and often better—than teens who lived with two married parents. DeLeire and Kalil concluded that the presence of a grandparent may be especially beneficial to low-income teens.

OVERCOMING THE STIGMA

Until the last quarter of the 20th century, children born to unmarried mothers were considered "illegitimate," and divorce was seen as a failure. But as divorce and births to unmarried mothers have become more common, single-parent families have come to be seen as one of many alternative family structures.

There are more than 11.6 million single-parent families in the United States; the great majority are headed by a female parent. Single parents face a host of challenges in raising their children alone. Yet most single parents provide their children not only with food, clothing, and shelter, but also with a supportive environment.

Many single parents rely on extended families and friends for emotional and social support; some turn to government assistance programs for help. The image of the welfare mom who sits at home and collects dollars is a myth. The truth is that most single parents work both within and outside the home.

See also: Day Care; Death in the Family; Divorce and Families; Family, The New; Family, The Traditional; Marriage and Family, Changes in; Teenage Parents

FURTHER READING

Baird, Craig. *A Complete Guide for Single Dads: Everything You Need to Know About Raising Healthy, Happy Children on Your Own.* Back-to-Basics. Ocala, Fla.: Atlantic Publishing Group Inc., 2010.

Chalkoun, Sandy. *Single Mother in Charge: How to Successfully Pursue Happiness.* Santa Barbara, Calif.: Praeger, 2010.

Price, Sharon. *Families & Change: Coping With Stressful Events and Transitions*. Thousand Oaks, Calif.: Sage Publications Inc., 2010.

■ STEPPARENTS

Stepparents are the spouses of one's parents by a subsequent marriage. The relationship between teens and stepparents is often turbulent. Some of the major challenges faced by stepparents are gaining respect, providing appropriate discipline and guidance, and negotiating their relationship with their new partner's ex-spouse.

GAINING RESPECT

Stepchildren are often reluctant participants in families created by a parent's remarriage. Children face several key tasks after a parent remarries. Children must adjust to the fact of their biological parent's remarriage, deal with possible changes in their own relationship with the biological parent, and form a relationship with a new stepparent, according to E. Mavis Hetherington, a leading researcher in stepfamily dynamics and professor of psychology at the University of California. Children may be disappointed or angry that a parent has remarried, and may resent the entry of another adult into the family.

Dealing with a new stepparent may be most difficult for teens, according to Hetherington. In a 1992 study published in *Monographs of the Society for Research in Child Development*, Hetherington and colleagues found that teens may feel that by accepting the new stepparent they are being disloyal to the noncustodial biological parent. These feelings may lead them to reject stepparents' efforts to extend friendship. In addition, Hetherington observes, teens are in the midst of their own transition from childhood to adulthood and dealing with the accompanying physical, social, emotional, intellectual, and behavioral changes. They are preparing to leave home and begin their own lives, becoming more independent and making decisions on their own. They are learning how to develop mature friendships and intimate relationships while maintaining close relationships with their parents and siblings. In stepfamilies, teens face the added task of negotiating a relationship with a person who is not quite a parent yet plays a fatherly or motherly role in their lives.

The vaguely defined role of the stepparent may add to the difficulties often experienced by stepparents and stepchildren. As sociologist Anne C. Jones notes in a study published by *Social Work* in April 2003, myths—unrealistic beliefs—about the "lesser" status of stepfamilies can cause problems in those families. Fairy tales and folklore abound with images of wicked stepmothers—images that may be difficult for even the most compassionate and caring stepmother to overcome. Jones notes that children in the United States grow up surrounded by fictional portraits of stepparents as abusive and dangerous. Neither are idealized stories about stepfamilies, such as television's *Brady Bunch,* helpful. According to Jones, these "one big happy family" stories create unrealistically high expectations that are likely to lead to frustration and disappointment.

Fact Or Fiction?

Stepmothers are cruel to their stepchildren.

The Facts: Stepmothers often do experience conflict with stepchildren, but not because they're the slave-driving, stepchild-hating stepmothers of Cinderella or Snow White nor the self-absorbed and disinterested stepmothers portrayed in television shows. Stepmothers simply tend to be more involved than stepfathers in their stepchildren's everyday lives. Many stepmothers quickly take on responsibilities, such as taking children to school and other activities and providing emotional support and discipline. The greater amount of time spent together creates more chances for conflict. However, it also provides an opportunity for a special bond to develop between stepmothers and stepchildren.

Many stepparents unrealistically expect their stepchildren to immediately offer them love, affection, and respect. Both stepfathers and stepmothers, hoping for a successful marriage, may try to gain immediate favor with their stepchildren. Yet, as Hetherington found in a 1999 study, *Coping with Divorce, Single Parenting, and Remarriage: A Risk and Resiliency Perspective,* stepchildren—especially stepdaughters—may meet stepparents' efforts with resistance and aversion. In turn, stepparents may withdraw, feel less close, and offer less warmth and guidance than biological parents in nonstepfamilies.

Q & A

Question: Should I love my stepmother?

Answer: When a parent remarries, many teens feel confused, conflicted about loyalties, angry, and even sad. Even if you don't feel negatively toward your new stepparent, you may not feel excited and happy about the changes she brings. You do not need to feel love toward your new stepmother right away. You may eventually develop a close, loving bond with her—or you may not. For now, be patient, treat her respectfully, and try to get to know her. Ask her if she would be willing to spend some time alone with you so you can talk about some of your feelings. If tempers keep flaring and you can't get along, your family may want to talk to a therapist.

Gender may affect interactions with teen stepchildren, as well as the teen's well-being. In 2003, the *Journal of Divorce and Remarriage* published a study on teens' self-esteem and their relationships with their biological parents and stepparents. Study author Ellen C. Berg, a professor of sociology at California State University, found that teens scored highest on measures of self-esteem when they felt closer to their biological mothers or stepmothers. The effect of closeness to stepfathers was not as great, leading Berg to suggest that feelings of closeness to the female parent with whom the teen lives may have the most impact on teens' self-esteem.

Biological parents often want their children to get along with their stepparents, which may lead to confusion about the true nature of the relationship between teens and stepparents. According to a study published in 2004 by the *Journal of Divorce and Remarriage,* biological parents and teens often perceive teens' relationships with their stepparents differently. The study, conducted by a research team led by Susan Silverberg Koerner of the University of Arizona, compared biological mothers' and teens' perceptions of the teens' relationship with the mothers' new partners. Of the 83 mother-daughter pairs, 47 had different perceptions of the teen-stepparent (or partner) relationship.

Mothers and daughters differed in their perceptions of three major areas: the quality of the relationship between the teen and the mother's new partner, the impact of the new partner on the family's life, and the impact of having a partner on the relationship between the mother and the teen. For instance, the mother often perceived the teen's relationship with the stepfather as "good" or "fine," while the teen felt uncomfortable or irritated by the mother's partner. In another common scenario, the mother acknowledged that problems had occurred early in the relationship but felt that things had been resolved, while the teen described the present relationship with the partner as "poor" or disliked the partner. In yet another variation, the mother focused on negative experiences between the teen and her partner while the teen described the partner (or his or her relationship with the partner) as "fine" or "good."

The researchers concluded that the differing perceptions of mothers and teens had a variety of causes. The mothers and teen may not have been communicating well, and they could have been holding back information or feelings from each other in an attempt to protect their relationship. Finally, the mothers and teens may have different investments in the relationship with the stepfathers. Mothers may hope that all will go smoothly, while teens may feel disloyal to their biological fathers if they easily accept the mother's new partner.

A 2008 study examined how stepchildren can feel "caught in the middle" between their parents' living in different households. Researchers found that when stepchildren did not feel caught in the middle it was related to higher levels of closeness within the family and their being centered within the family. In 2010, researchers for the *Journal of Research on Adolescence* conducted a longitudinal study of parental disruption with 236 early adolescent children and their mothers. The findings showed that greater conflict between the mother and biological child was increased with the presence of half-siblings. This effect was not found with the entrance of the stepfathers into the home.

DISCIPLINE

As a responsible adult, the stepparent is accountable for the well-being, guidance, and protection of children. Yet conflicts over child discipline top the list of relationship problems for many remarried couples.

In 1971, psychologist Diana Baumrind described three parenting styles—authoritative, permissive, and authoritarian. According to Baumrind, parents who use an authoritative style are firm in their decisions, clear in their guidelines, keep track of their children's activities, and have relatively high expectations for their children. Authoritative parents also offer their children warmth and affection, reason with their children, and encourage children to reach agreements through verbal exchanges. Permissive parents tend to respond to children's needs; they are less apt to punish and expect less of their children. Authoritarian parents tend to be highly demanding, expect unquestioning obedience, make decisions without explanations, and offer less warmth.

Psychologists and sociologists still use these categories to describe types of parenting, although more recent research, such as a study of parenting styles published by *Child Development* in 1992, suggests that parents often use a combination of different styles. The 1992 study, which was conducted by researchers from the Department of Psychology at Temple University, was one of many that supported Baumrind's finding that children tend to fare best when parents use an authoritative style. The Temple University researcher found that authoritative parenting leads to better school performance and school engagement among teens. According to Baumrind, adults who were reared in authoritative households tend to have a lively, happy disposition, feel self-confident about their ability to master tasks, regulate their emotions well, have well-developed social skills, and are less rigid about gender-typed traits.

A study published by the journal *Communication Quarterly* suggests that the effects of parenting styles may be more complex between stepparents and stepchildren. Tamara Golish of the University of Nebraska interviewed 115 teens and young adults who lived in stepfamilies. She asked them about the parenting styles used by their stepparents. Golish found that more authoritarian stepparenting tended to increase the tendency of stepchildren to avoid talking about important topics with stepfamily members. When stepparents were more permissive or more authoritative, children were more open about their feelings and less likely to avoid difficult topics. Teens who perceived their stepparents parenting style as authoritarian were generally less satisfied with their relationship with their stepparent. When stepparents showed low or high degrees of permissiveness, teens were also less satisfied; in contrast, teens felt moderately satisfied with moderately permissive stepparents. Teens were more accepting of stepparents who were authoritative.

In 2010, the *Journal of Genetic Psychology* published findings that examined parenting style and the healthy development of adolescents. The results indicated that authoritative parenting style during adolescence decreased adolescent depression and increased adolescent sense of self-esteem. The authors concluded that authoritative parenting made for healthy self-development as adolescents grow into adulthood.

TO ADOPT OR NOT TO ADOPT?

Stepparents often provide stepchildren with tangible support such as food, clothing, and housing, and many form deep emotional bonds with stepchildren. But a stepparent is not legally required to support a spouse's children nor does the stepparent have parental rights. Marrying a child's custodial parent does not give an adult legal rights to the child. The stepparent has no legal ties to the child if the marriage ends, or the biological parent dies or becomes incapacitated. For this reason, many remarried couples choose to have the stepparent legally adopt his or her spouse's biological children.

Adoption of a stepchild signifies a practical commitment on the part of the stepparent. The stepparent takes on parental responsibilities to nurture, provide for, and protect the child and releases the non-custodial parent of parental responsibilities. Stepparent adoption also signifies an emotional commitment to the marriage and the new ·family. For these and other reasons, stepparent adoption is the most common type of adoption in the United States.

In most cases, the noncustodial parent must consent to the adoption. In consenting, the noncustodial parent gives up all parental rights and is relieved of parental responsibilities, including child support. Parental rights include the right to visit and make decisions about medical treatment or education. If the noncustodial parent refuses to consent to the adoption, the adoption cannot take place except in specific circumstances. Some states allow parental rights to be terminated if the noncustodial parent is absent or has not exercised parental rights such as visiting or communicating with the child. In most states, termination of parental rights is allowed when a parent has willfully failed to support the child or has abandoned the child for a certain length of time, usually a year. **Abandonment** usually means that the absent parent hasn't communicated with or financially supported the child. In 49 states, older children must also consent to their own adoption. In most states, children age 12 or older must consent to their own adoption. In Puerto Rico, a child age 10 or older must consent.

Stepchild adoption can have great emotional and financial impact on the family, especially if the noncustodial parent is alive, in frequent contact with the child, and paying child support. Children may feel that they must divide their attention and loyalty between their adoptive stepfather and biological father. After the adoption, the noncustodial parent no longer has the legal right to spend time with the child, known as **visitation rights.** On the other hand, adoption may signify stability and security to children, who may feel uncertain about their parent's remarriage. In general, the less contact children have with their noncustodial parent, the more likely it is that step-parent adoption will be to the benefit of the family. The family's economic circumstances may also dictate whether adoption is a good choice. If the noncustodial parent is paying child support on a regular basis, the loss of that income should be taken into account when considering stepparent adoption.

DEALING WITH THE OTHER PARENT

Dealing with a new spouse's former partner may be one of the most difficult aspects of a stepparent's life. Stepparents can easily become caught in a web of angry feelings between their new spouse, stepchildren, and the noncustodial parent. When ex-spouses do not get along well, the relationship between stepparents and stepchildren may be strained.

On the other hand, when stepparents are able to build positive relationships with their spouse's ex-partner, children may benefit, as suggested in a study published by the *Journal of Marriage and the Family* in February 2004. The study was authored by William Marsiglio, a sociologist at the University of Florida. Marsiglio examined the actions and attitudes that allowed stepfathers to develop fatherlike relationships with their stepchildren and to "claim" those children as their own. He interviewed 36 stepfathers at length for the study. He found that stepfathers tended to use either cooperative or competitive approaches in response to biological fathers' involvement. Stepfathers who used a cooperative approach claimed their stepchildren as their own while acknowledging that the biological father was an important person, and another father figure, in the child's life. Stepfathers who used a competitive approach saw the biological father as a competitor who did not have anything to do with their desire and ability to claim their stepchildren as their own. When stepfathers used a cooperative approach, stepfamilies were better able to see themselves as a cohesive group.

Likewise, a study published in 2001 by the *Journal of Marriage and the Family* suggests that children benefit when they have warm relationships with both biological and stepfathers. The study, "When Children Have Two Fathers: Effects of Relationships with Stepfathers and Non-custodial Fathers on Adolescent Outcomes," was authored by University of Nebraska sociologists Lynne White and Joan G. Gilbreth. White and Gilbreth surveyed 189 children, as well as their mothers and stepfathers, about the effects of children's relationships with biological and stepfathers on their well-being. White and Gilbreth found that children who felt strong and affectionate bonds with their stepfather and biological mother had fewer behavior problems. More children who lived in stepfamilies said they had good relationships with their biological, noncustodial fathers than did children who lived in single-parent families. According to White and Gilbreth, their results support the idea that children benefit when stepfathers are perceived as a second father—as opposed to a substitute father.

According to a 2010 study in the journal *Fathering,* shared communication and emotional closeness between stepfathers and children reduce alcohol problems in children. This positive effect of the father-child relationship on a child's involvement with alcohol was determined to be even stronger than the effect of the same mother-child relationship.

These and other studies suggest that stepfamily members may benefit when families are able to establish a **parenting coalition** in which the divorced and remarried biological parents and the stepparents cooperate in rearing their biological children and stepchildren. Children have contact with both of their parents and with their stepparents. In this type of cooperative arrangement, the children's needs, as well as the needs of the adults, can be met more easily. The sharing of parenting responsibilities reduces the burden on parents and ensures that children are not used as messengers to carry parents' anger back and forth. Children are better able to perceive the stepparent as another important adult in their lives, not as a person who is interfering with their relationship with their parent. Parenting coalitions minimize power struggles between households and recognize stepparents as important people in an ever-changing family.

Stepfamilies face several tasks, including the establishment of relationships between stepchildren and stepparents. Stepparents who expect stepchildren to love and respect them immediately are likely to be disappointed. Discipline is a common problem between stepparents and stepchildren. Stepparents who use an authoritative parenting style are most likely to gain the respect of their stepchildren. Stepparent adoption can have both positive and negative effects on the stepfamily. While adoption can represent a commitment to the spouse's children and ensure they are cared for if a biological parent dies, it may also mean loss of child support payments and lessen children's contact with the noncustodial biological parent. Children may benefit when their biological and stepparents see themselves as sharing, rather than competing, in their parental roles.

See also: Adoption; Arguments and the Family; Divorce and Families; Families, Blended; Families, Divided; Family, The New; Marriage and Family, Changes in

FURTHER READING

Penton, John. *Yours, Mine and Hours: Relationship Skills for Blended Families.* Seattle, Wash.: BookSurge Publishing, 2007.

Wednesday, Martin. *Stepmonster: A New Look at Why Real Stepmothers Think, Feel, and Act the Way We Do.* New York: Houghton Mifflin Harcourt, 2010.

■ TEENAGE PARENTS

Teenage parents are those under the age of 20. Parenthood is a life-changing event for a person of any age, but for teen parents, the responsibilities of rearing a child may interfere with their own growth into adulthood. How many teens in the United States are parents, and what challenges do they and their children face?

FACTS AND FIGURES IN AMERICA

Between 1991 and 2005, the birthrate for American teenagers fell by 34 percent according to the National Center for Health Statistics. However, the same group found that between 2005 and 2006, the rate increased by 3 percent. The birthrate for babies born to girls 14 and under continues to fall, but the rate for girls ages 15 to 19 increased from 40.5 live births per 1,000 girls to 41.9 live births per 1,000 girls in 2006. Teen birthrates were the lowest in the North and Northeast regions on the United States and highest in the South and Southwest regions. However, overall, the report found that the average age of a new mother remains 25 years old.

This same report explained that, in 2006, more than 1.6 million babies were born to unmarried mothers. This is the highest number in U.S. history. More than 80 percent of the babies born to teenage mothers in 2006 entered families of unmarried parents. Also, 25 percent of babies born to unmarried women under the age of 25 did not have a father's name listed on the birth certificate. Utah and New

U.S. Birthrates for Teens Aged 15–19, by Race

Race

■ 1991 ■ 2000 ■ 2005 ■ 2006

The birthrate for teenagers in all racial groups in the United States has decreased steadily since 1991. During 1991–2005, for Non-Hispanic black teens aged 15–19, for example, the birthrate dropped from 118 per every 1,000 females in 1991 to 61 births in 2005–a 48 percent decrease. Rates increased slightly (3 to 4 percent) for all groups, except Asian or Pacific Islanders, in 2006 due only to a 2 percent increase in the number of U.S. teenagers.

Source: *National Vital Statistics Reports*, Number 7, Centers for Disease Control and Prevention, 2009.

Hampshire reported the lowest number of births to unmarried mothers while Louisiana, Mississippi, and New Mexico reported the highest.

Teen fathers are likely to be older than teen mothers, sometimes significantly. Research completed by Denise Hines and David Finkelhor explains that statutory relationships that involve a younger girl and a much older man have a higher risk for a teen pregnancy, for the mother to have to raise the baby as a single parent, and for other psychosocial problems for the teen mother. In addition, the researchers found that almost 70 percent of unmarried adolescent girls who have a sexual partner six years or older will become pregnant. This is almost four times more than those who have a relationship with a partner only two years older.

The Alan Guttmacher Institute (AGI), a nonprofit research organization focused on sexual and reproductive health issues, reported in 2010 that approximately 14 percent of teens who become pregnant miscarry, and 27 percent end their pregnancies through abortion. Latina teens are most likely, and African-American teens least likely, to have a pregnancy that ends in a live birth. Among teens who give birth, more than 96 percent keep their babies; less than 4 percent make an adoption plan for their infants.

Poverty and teen parents
An analysis of public policy issues surrounding teen parenthood was published in 2003 as part of the collection *All Our Families: New Policies for a New Century.* Author Jane Mauldon, a public policy researcher at the University of California–Berkeley, describes poverty and teen parenthood as "twinned experiences." Mauldon cites statistics from the AGI that show teens from low-income families are nine times more likely to give birth to a child than are teens from higher-income families. While 38 percent of teens live in low-income families, they account for 83 percent of teen births. This may be because low-income teens are more likely to start having sex at a young age, less likely to use contraception, and less likely to have abortions, according to Mauldon. In addition, the National Campaign to Prevent Teen and Unplanned Pregnancy completed a report that finds that the cost to federal, state, and local taxpayers for teen pregnancy is $1.9 billion.

Mauldon suggests that poverty is both a cause and result of teen pregnancy. She suggests that for teenage women living in low-income families and communities, motherhood may offer a sort of "pseudo-adulthood" that allows the teen to assume meaningful responsibilities—such as caring for a child—and status. At the same time, she can remain dependent on her family and, often, the government, so she is not completely cut off from her support systems. Teens who have not succeeded in other parts of their lives, such as school, may believe that motherhood provides a chance to show that they have mastered important skills. Mauldon also points out that many teenage mothers are emotionally needy, often because they have experienced abuse, neglect, or molestation. AGI research shows that 10 percent of young women between the ages of 18 and 24 who had sex for the first time before the age of 20 reported it to be involuntary.

A survey by the National Campaign to Prevent Teen and Unplanned Pregnancy reported that teen parents represent every socioeconomic and demographic category, and in fact, almost half of teen parents in the United States come from households that are at or 200 percent above the federal poverty line. In fact, 70 percent of teen parents were raised by two parents. However, the same organization found that the rate of unplanned pregnancies had increased among women in poverty and those with less education. Still, statistics show that half of *all* pregnancies are unplanned.

QUALITY OF LIFE

The socioeconomic status of parents, especially teen parents, has an impact on the quality of life for the child. Twenty-five percent of all teen mothers will go on welfare within the first three years of their child's life. One area of income that is usually not supplemented is in the form of child support. Nearly 80 percent of fathers to children born to teen mothers do not marry the mother, and these fathers pay less than 800 dollars annually for child support, primarily because they are living in poverty themselves. The National Campaign to Prevent Teen and Unplanned Pregnancy writes that if a child is born to a teen mom, who is not married to the father, and who dropped out of high school, the child is nine times more likely to grow up in poverty than a child who grows up in a household that did not have those factors present.

Because the same organization finds that only half of teen mothers gain a high school diploma, poverty is a real possibility for the children of teen parents. In fact, one of the leading reasons why a teen drops out of high school is due to parenthood. Once a student drops out, it is not likely that she or he will return to school to complete a degree. Less than 2 percent of mothers who have a child before the age of 18 will complete a college degree before they are 30 years old.

EDUCATION AND TEEN PARENTS

Interestingly, this trend of dropping out actually can be seen in the children of teen moms as well. The same organization found that only two-thirds of children born to teen moms will graduate from high school as opposed to the 81 percent of kids born to parents who had their children later in life. Research also shows that teens that fail in school are more likely to be teen parents. The National Campaign to Prevent Teen and Unplanned pregnancy has also found that simply planning to attend college following high school is associated with lower teen pregnancy risk. Even just being more involved in school-related activities has shown an association with a lower risk of teen pregnancy. Overall, studies show that staying in school and gaining an education can help to prevent teen pregnancy.

CHALLENGES FOR TEEN PARENTS

While the demands of parenting are great at any age, teen parents often face additional challenges. Teens are at a critical stage in the development of their identities. How will they move out of their family home and create a home of their own? What occupation will they choose? What values will they live their lives by? Early parent-hood can interfere with these developmental tasks. The teen parent has little time for dating, friendships, schooling, and career choices. Most teen parents have not yet completed their education, have little money, and lack job skills. They often must take on part-time work to pay for the expenses of having a child.

TEENS SPEAK

I'm a Teenage Mom

My mother was the one who first recognized that I was pregnant. I think I already knew, but I denied it until the day my mother said to me, "Marcia, I think you're pregnant." She took me to see her obstetrician, a physician who specializes in delivering babies. The doctor ran more tests and confirmed that I was almost four months pregnant.

That's when reality hit me: I was 15 years old, about to have a baby, and alone. My baby's father didn't want anything to do with me. He had been lead quarterback on the football team at my high school, the guy everybody wanted to date. When he wanted to have sex, I said yes because I thought it meant he loved me. But he broke up with me about a week after I had sex with him.

My labor was horrible. It lasted almost 30 hours, and it was the most painful experience I have ever had. The doctor said it was difficult because my pelvis was so small. When it was all over, I had a little girl. I named her Sara.

Sara is six months old now. She often wakes up in the middle of the night crying, and I can't figure out what she wants. It's not like having a doll, or even a dog. I can't leave her alone. I'm usually exhausted: I can't remember the last time I slept more than four hours. I rarely go out with my friends anymore, partly because I'm too tired by Friday night, and partly because my parents won't watch her on weekends. As far as dating anyone, forget it. Everyone at my school knows that I'm a mom, and no guys want to take on that responsibility. Besides, what teenage guy wants to go on a date with a baby stroller?

Before I got pregnant, I planned to become a veterinarian. But that's not going to happen now, at least not until Sara is almost grown. Still, I'm determined to finish school and get a decent job so I can move out of my parents' house someday. I may even be able to go to college, but it will be a lot harder than if I didn't have to care for a child. I wish I'd waited until I was older to become a mom.

Several studies have examined the connection between teen parenthood and psychological problems such as an overwhelming feeling of sadness and grief, known as **depression**. Recent findings published in the *Journal of Youth and Adolescence* explain that teen mothers are especially prone to depression because they represent two categories of people more susceptible to depression: adolescents and mothers. Depression that begins shortly after giving birth is known as **postpartum depression.** The authors Elaine Eshbaugh, Jacques Lempers, and Gayle Luze point out some factors that have been known to contribute to depression: income and education levels, having or not having someone to talk to or lend support, and even the worry of weight gain. All of these concerns can have a major effect on the mental health of a teen mother.

However, research shows that the mental health status of teen moms can vary with educational accomplishments and even with age. The authors wrote that younger adolescent mothers may experience more depression than older adolescent mothers because of the internal growing process that the young woman is experiencing on top of her attempt to raise a healthy child. All of these pressures are in the face of a community stigma that still exists for unwed, teenage mothers, which, the researchers point out, can compound the young woman's depression.

In a recent study on the trauma and depression levels of 28 teenage mothers, researchers Cheryl Anderson and Teena McGuinness reported that they believe that teen moms may be more prone to post-traumatic stress disorder (PTSD) as a result of the childbirth experience. They explain that while pregnancy, labor, and delivery can be difficult for every mother, they can be especially hard for a teen mother who may not have the necessary support system or proper knowledge. They also wrote that postpartum depression runs among teen mothers, especially those without social support or with family conflict. In fact, the researchers claim that the rate of depression for teen moms was almost twice as high as that of adult moms.

Teen parenthood often affects the teen's own parents, especially if the teen continues to live at home. According to an article by Elaine Eshbaugh, a researcher in the Department of Family Studies from the University of Northern Iowa, several state assistance programs in place for teen mothers require them to co-reside with an adult caretaker. While this is meant to provide the teens with an opportunity to finish school and obtain care and support, it can lead to unintended consequences for the household. Dr. Eshbaugh found several studies that support the notion that co-residence for teen mothers during the first few years of their child's life led the mothers to be less dependent on welfare programs in the future and more successful with their education. However, other studies have suggested that a teen mother who lives alone with her child is more likely to have more parent-child interaction and even more affection. The article even mentions previous research that found the role of the teen parent and the grandparent can become blurred in the eyes of the child.

Teenage mothers and their families bear the brunt of teen parenthood, but teen fathers are also affected. Teen fathers who choose to honor their parenthood because of a sense of responsibility or because of affection and commitment to the mother or child may find their lives drastically altered. They may decide to marry the teen mother, which often means changing their plans for completing their education, choosing an occupation, and pursuing other life goals. The father may be met with resentment and anger from the family of the teen mother. In addition, at a time when his financial resources are few and uncertain, the teen father may be called upon to provide financial assistance to the teen mother and his child, known as **child support.**

Q & A

Question: I'm a teen dad. My son's mother and I are no longer dating, but I want to be a part of my son's life. How can I?

Answer: If you haven't done so already, establish that you are the father of the child, called paternity. You can do this at a hospital or at the county birth records office. If you don't establish your paternity, you will have no legal right to visitation or custody of the child. Next, create a child support agreement with the mother of your child. How much can you reasonably pay? Quitting school to work full-time is a bad idea. Instead, consider staying in school and getting a part-time job. Finally, visit, write, call, or e-mail your son as often as you can. Your son needs your emotional support—attention, care, affection, and love—as well as his mother's.

Teenage marriages are rare and generally unstable. Census Bureau data show that in 2009, only 2.1 percent of teens age 15 to 19 had ever been married, compared to 11 percent in 1975. In 2006, researchers Barbara Dafoe Whitehead and Marline Pearson helped to write *Making a Love Connection: Teen Relationships, Pregnancy, and Marriage,* a manual on the new sequencing occurring in the lives of teens. They found that over time, the order in which teens have children, get married, and have sex is no longer the same as it was in the past. In fact, they explain that some teens today do not even see the three life events as having a natural connection, while in the past, it was much more definitive that marriage was followed by pregnancy.

Fact Or Fiction?

If teen parents married, they and their children would have fewer problems.

The Facts: There are three compelling reasons why marriage does not provide long-term stability to teen parents. First, teens who marry are more likely to divorce than are young adults. Second, married teen mothers are actually less likely to finish high school than those who remain unmarried, making it less likely that they will be able to find a job that pays well. Third, most teen fathers (and young adult partners of teen mothers) have low educational levels, little work experience, and few job skills. Thus, although early marriage may provide a short-term solution to poverty and the challenges of single-parenting, for most teen parents, early marriage may really be a route into long-term underemployment and fewer life options.

The researchers performed analyses of data from Fragile Families, a nationally representative sample of births in metropolitan areas in the United States. The results from the Fragile Families study showed that raising children in nonmarital households has risen to 40 percent of all births in 2007 as compared to only 6 percent of all births in the 1960s. The research also proved that unmarried couples usually break up within a few years of their child's birth. Additionally, most teen parents will not last even a few years with their partner. Instead, serial cohabitation is more common among teenage, unmarried birth mothers. In fact, research by Deborah Graefe of the Population Institute of Pennsylvania State University found that unmarried women who have children will forever change the course of all of their future relationships and marriage opportunities. Teens who do marry are not likely to stay married. One-third of marriages that occur before the woman is 18 end in divorce within five years. Almost half will end in 10 years.

STAYING IN SCHOOL

Less than 40 percent of teenage mothers graduate from high school, and far fewer go on to college. Most drop out because of the demands of parenting, the need to work, and a lack of time. While peers are going to football games and experimenting with relationships, teen mothers are changing diapers and warming baby bottles when they're not working to make ends meet. Even the most popular of teens often find that their popularity wanes. Teen fathers often find themselves working to help support their children, whether or not they are involved in parenting.

Many states have programs designed to help teen parents stay in school. For instance, in 2006, the state of Colorado began using some federal dollars for a Responsible Fatherhood initiative with the help of different faith-based organizations and community centers. Several of the programs that received funding are aimed at preparing teen fathers to be responsible and active. Many high schools offer programs for teen mothers that include on-site day care services, early childhood education, and other support services. Such programs recognize that teens face special challenges in both pregnancy and parenthood.

A few schools, such as Milwaukee's Lady Pitts School Age Parent Center, focus exclusively on helping pregnant and parenting teens navigate both school and parenthood. All of the students at Lady Pitts are pregnant or parenting teens. Other programs are designed to help pregnant teens to gain the job and parenting skills they need. Most have three goals: to help teen parents complete high school, improve their job skills and employability, and to promote the health and development of teens' children. For instance, California's "Cal-Learn" program, which serves parenting teens who receive welfare, combines guidance with financial incentives. Each teen parent is assigned a "case manager" who helps her to organize school, child care, health care, and other needs. Teens receive an extra $100 for every report card that shows they're making satisfactory progress in school. If they drop out, or if they receive a report card showing unsatisfactory progress, $100 is deducted from their welfare check. Upon graduation, they receive a $500 bonus. University of California, Berkeley investigators evaluated the program in 2000. The program increased graduation rates among teens who had dropped out of school but returned to earn their GEDs. By their 20th birthday, nearly half (47 percent) of the teens in the program had graduated or earned their GED, in comparison to 33 percent of those not enrolled in the program.

Programs to help teen fathers are also becoming more common. Researchers from the Department of Family and Child Ecology at Michigan State University looked at six adolescent fathers and the role of a parenting class. These young men also were in a juvenile probation program for criminal offenses. Each of the fathers successfully completed a parenting program aimed at teen dads. The teens expressed a gradual acceptance of and excitement about fatherhood. The results of the study also showed that the participants felt challenged and sometimes angry over their new role. However, they also reported that they felt joy once they committed to being good fathers. Still, many of the teens in the study reported they did not have the same relationship with the mother of their baby as they did before the birth. However, despite this, the participants in this study said that they would like to maintain a good relationship with the mother for the sake of their child. After successfully completing the parenting course for teen dads, most of the participants, the researchers found, were actively trying to be better fathers.

HOW DO KIDS FARE?

The children of teen parents are at risk in many areas of their lives, and this risk may begin during the teen's pregnancy. Studies such as one published in 2007 by the *Journal of International Epidemiology* suggest that one reason children of teen parents have more problems may have more to do with poverty and lack of prenatal care. According to a 2010 report by the AGI, teens are less likely than adult mothers to receive medical care during pregnancy, known as **prenatal** care. Pregnant teens are also more likely to experiment with drugs, alcohol, tobacco, use caffeine, and eat a nutritionally poor diet during pregnancy. All of these behaviors increase the risk of damage to the **fetus**—the unborn baby from the eighth week after fertilization to birth.

Teenage mothers are at greater risk of giving birth to low birth weight babies—infants weighing less than 2,500 grams, or 5.5 pounds, at birth—than are women age 24 to 35. Data from a 2007 study in the *Journal of International Epidemiology* revealed that in all of the teenage groups of birth outcomes that were researched, each one was associated with preterm delivery and low birth weight. Low birth weight is associated with childhood health problems, frequent hospitalization, and other complications. It is not clear whether this is due to the age of the mother or to lack of prenatal care, lack of knowledge about pregnancy, or other factors associated with the low-income status of many teen parents.

Women who smoke are twice as likely to have a low birth weight baby than those who do not. A study in *International Family Planning Perspectives* in 2008 also explains that even low levels of tobacco use among young women of childbearing age has not only a negative health impact on the woman but also that smoking during a pregnancy is linked to preterm delivery, low birth weight, and other problems with the baby. Education level also affects the probability of having a low birth weight baby. In 2009, authors of an article in the *Journal of Health Economics* found a significant association between parental education and a baby's birth weight. The researchers found that the higher the education, the better the birth weight.

But race and socioeconomic class may only partly affect the chance of a teen mother giving birth to a low birth weight infant. In 2009, research was published in the *Perspectives on Sexual and Reproductive*

Health that showed that teen mothers are more likely to have a baby with a low birth weight, no matter if they come from a higher income bracket or obtain education. The researchers discovered that women under the age of 16 who became pregnant with their second child would still be prone to delivering babies with low birth weight. The paper showed that teen mothers have babies with lower birth weights than their older counterparts.

Studies have consistently shown that children of teen parents may not acquire language, learning, and thinking abilities as quickly as those of adult mothers. According to research in 2009 from the University of Pittsburgh School of Medicine, children who are born to teen mothers are at more risk for physical and cognitive problems than babies born to adult mothers. The researchers found the children born to teen and adolescent girls have poor growth outcomes. Additionally, they reported that children born to teenagers had higher rates of intellectual, language, and socio-emotional delays than children born to older women.

Several studies have shown that teen mothers' depression may lead to problems for their children. Findings from an article published in 2008 in the *American Journal of Psychiatry* indicate that children of depressed mothers are more prone to disorders themselves. The authors explained that while the developmental stages of children will vary, those born to depressed mothers have been associated with more behavior and anxiety disorders. Many times these issues begin before puberty, with an onset of major depression commonly occurring in early adolescence. The authors noted that substance abuse disorders can occur in children born to depressed mothers when the child hits late adolescence or early adulthood.

In 2007, the *Journal of School Health* conducted a study of teen mothers in an urban high school to determine outcomes of the mother following a parenting support program and a school-based child care center. The results showed that of the 65 adolescent mothers in the study, 33 percent were depressed and almost 40 percent had experienced some kind of homelessness. The mothers did not have much of a network for social support and reported negative life events in the past year. The researchers also looked at the developmental and health outcomes of the participants' children. They found seven of the children to have developmental delays. The results indicated that participation in the parenting support program as well as access to the school-based child care were positive to both the mother's emotional and mental well-being and the development and health of the child. In short, the teen mothers in the study benefited from outside help and support in the growth of their babies.

Researchers in 2007, publishing in the journal *Perspectives on Sexual and Reproductive Health,* looked at the indicators for second births to teen mothers and found one of the biggest predictors to be lack or perceived lack of support. In fact, the adolescents in the study who reported a second birth also said that they were not close to their mother and/or they did not feel that they had family support. This theme is expressed throughout much research, namely that the disconnection from a teen's family can cause the young mother more stress and anxiety than is normal and greater levels of depression. Unfortunately, the article also noted that the teen respondents going through a repeat pregnancy reported that they had been hit by their boyfriend or husband in the three months after the birth. In addition, the authors revealed that the adolescent mothers who said that their peer relationships and support were from other teen mothers were more likely to have a second birth while still less than 19 years old.

Although the behavioral and emotional problems of children of teen parents may stem partly from their parents' inadequate parenting skills, many teen parents can improve those skills. A study at Yale University in 2007 looked at school-based parenting programs for teen parents and their children. Researchers compared these parenting programs to school-based health centers and found them to be great models of service for vulnerable youth. The academic researchers discovered that one of the major strengths of a school-based parenting program is that there is daily contact between the health and educational specialist and the young mother and child. The results of the study showed that because the classes created a daily involvement at the school, the young mothers were able to stay connected to their children in the child care center and to remain active in school. They were also given access to health care, especially reproductive care, and supplied parental role models to watch. This particular school-based program even assisted those young mothers who dropped out of school so that they too could get the support they needed.

After dramatic declines in teen pregnancy from 1991 to 2005, the teen birthrate in the United States actually began to increase in 2006 and 2007. Research suggests that the higher rates of teen pregnancies and births in the United States, as compared to Europe, may be due to a lower contraception use among sexually active teens, according to the AGI. The great majority of teen parents are single and come from low-income families. While 38 percent of teens live in low-income families, they account for 83 percent of teen births. Because teens are at a critical stage in the development of their own identities, the demands of parenting may be overwhelming for them. Less than 50 percent of teenage mothers graduate from high school, and far fewer go on to college. Teen mothers who drop out of school before becoming pregnant are least likely to finish school. Almost half of teen mothers experience depression after the birth of their babies, which may contribute to the behavioral, emotional, and intellectual problems often seen in children of teen mothers. Children of teen parents may have fewer developmental problems when teen parents develop their parenting skills and enlist the support of family members.

Having a child during teenage years can be a handicap; much depends on how the teen parents chose to cope with the situation. Many teen mothers and fathers finish school, attend college, gain work experience, and go on to have satisfying careers and family lives. Support programs that offer training in self-esteem, relationships, health care, birth control, parenting, life skills, decision making, and goal setting have been shown to be effective in helping teen parents negotiate the demands of early parenthood.

See also: Adoption; Arguments and the Family; Birth Order and Psychology; Day Care; Family, The New; Puberty and Sexual Development; Single-Parent Families; Teens in Trouble

FURTHER READING

Kiselica, Mark S. *When Boys Become Parents: Adolescent Fatherhood in America.* Piscataway, N.J.: Rutgers University Press, 2008.

Lyon, Maureen E., and Christina Brede Antoniades. *My Teen Has Had Sex, Now What Do I Do?: How to Help Teens Make Safe, Sensible, Self-Reliant Choices When They've Already Said "Yes."* Beverly, Mass.: Rockport Publishers, 2009.

Spilsbury, Louise, and Mike Gordon. *Me, Myself and I: All About Sex and Puberty.* Hauppauge, N.Y.: Barron's Educational Series, 2010.

■ TEENS IN TROUBLE

Adolescence is a period of transition from childhood to adulthood. It is a time of physical, emotional, and behavioral changes. Understandably, many teens (and their parents) wonder whether their feelings, attitudes, and behaviors are "normal." Are they cause for concern?

The American Academy of Child and Adolescent Psychiatry (AACAP) maintains that most teens find it difficult to deal with peer pressure, dating, their own emerging sexuality, issues of independence, and anxiety over schoolwork. Many are also dealing with violence at home or in their community, the availability of alcohol and illegal drugs, and depression.

When adolescents face such serious issues, family life is likely to be affected. Experts at the AACAP note that parents and professionals sometimes fail to identify the emotional and behavioral problems affecting teens. Yet if left untreated, these problems can lead to more serious problems. Early identification of adolescents who need special attention is important.

PHYSICAL HEALTH

Most adolescents are physically healthy. Yet large numbers of teens struggle with health issues related to unplanned pregnancy, sexually transmitted diseases, and violence.

The National Campaign to Prevent Teen Pregnancy notes that the United States has higher rates of teen pregnancy and births than other western countries. About 30 percent of young women become pregnant at least once before they reach the age of 20. The U.S. Teenage Pregnancy Statistics with Comparative Statistics for Women reports nearly 1 million teen pregnancies each year. Eight in 10 of these pregnancies are unplanned pregnancies, with 79 percent occurring to unmarried teens.

In a research study about the influence of families on teen pregnancy, the National Campaign to Prevent Teen Pregnancy found that teens say that parents have the greatest influence on their decisions about dating and relationships. Other studies seem to confirm those findings.

In a 2007 study, researchers Ronny Shtarkshall, John Santelli, and Jennifer Hirsch found that the role of fostering sexual knowledge and health in adolescents belongs to both parents and educators. They found that parents should be encouraged to explain the social, cultural, and religious values of intimate and sexual relationship, but that health and education professionals may be suited to explain more about sexuality and the related social skills. However, the authors admit that the two groups should work together and be invested in what a child is hearing from the other side. They felt that a combination of school-sponsored sexual education coupled with the moral consequences and issues coming from parents will allow a teen to have better sexual conduct and overall sexual health.

Sexually transmitted diseases (STDs) are acquired through intimate sexual contact with someone who is already infected with the disease. Every year, more than 13 million people become infected with STDs. According to the Alan Guttmacher Institute, a nonprofit research center focusing on sexual and reproductive health, one in four sexually active teens becomes infected with an STD every year. In 2010, only 35 of the 50 states, in addition to the District of Columbia, had mandatory sexually transmitted infection and HIV education. Only 18 of these states also required discussion about contraception. Common STDs are chlamydia, gonorrhea, genital warts, and herpes. According to the National Campaign to Prevent Teen Pregnancy, teens with strong ties to their parents and a stable family life are less likely to become sexually active early, therefore decreasing exposure to STDs.

Violence is yet another major health problem for teens. The Centers for Disease Control and Prevention reported in 2008 that almost one in four women in the United States will experience violence by a current or former spouse or boyfriend during their lifetime. Many people think that violence within a relationship occurs only between married persons. Yet experts define domestic violence to include any violence—including physical, verbal, and emotional abuse—between people who are dating, regardless of their sexual orientation. Abusive behavior is any act aimed at hurting or controlling another person. A violent relationship is about power and control and means more than being hit by a person who says they love or care about the victim.

The National Council on Crime and Delinquency Focus found in 2008 that one in three adolescent girls in the United States is a victim of abuse from a dating partner. This can be physical, emotional, or even verbal. This number is higher than any other rate of violence against youth. Additional research, *Tween and Teen Dating Violence and Abuse Study,* reported in 2008 that one in five "tweens" aged 11 to 14 were victims of dating violence with almost 50 percent claiming to have a friend who is verbally abused.

When teens are abused (whether the abuse comes from within the family or from a relationship outside the family), the effects are similar. Those effects include eating and sleeping disturbances, poor school performance, and difficulties with relationships at home or at school. Some teens may become depressed and even suicidal.

Q & A

Question: If teens witness violence within the family, are they at higher risk to become victims of dating violence?

Answer: The Family Violence Prevention Fund creates training manuals to help families understand how domestic violence can harm children. According to the organization, millions of children witness domestic violence every year, and this can be dangerous to them even if they are not abused or neglected directly.

Experts theorize that because teens are formulating their own ideas about relationships by watching the relationships of their parents, they may not have the best models on which to base a healthy relationship.

EMOTIONAL HEALTH

Teens often experience stress at school or at home, worry about their family's financial problems, or deal with a wide variety of fears related to growing up. For some teenagers, their parents' divorce, the formation of a new family with stepparents and step-siblings, or moving to a new community can be very emotional and can intensify typical issues of adolescence.

Teens need adult guidance to understand the emotional and physical changes they are experiencing. For some, managing these complex feelings is overwhelming. The American Association for Child and Adolescent Psychiatry claims that approximately five percent of children and adolescents experience depression. Recent surveys indicate that as many as one in five teens may suffer from clinical depression. **Depression** is more than just feeling down or blue about something that went wrong during the day. There are two types of depression. The first is called major depression, dysthymia, or reactive depression. It is the inability to interact with friends and family and even hope that things will get better with time. The second type is called bipolar disorder or manic depression. Those who are diagnosed with this condition don't feel happy one minute and sad the next. Instead they have times when they become so overexcited that they may become reckless and times they feel so sad that they may become suicidal. The highs are very high and the lows are very low.

Depression can be difficult to diagnose in teens because of the many myths about moody adolescents. Even teens do not always understand the significance or depth of their own depressed feelings.

The National Mental Health Association claims that some teens feel so depressed that they consider ending their lives. Suicide is the third leading cause of death among adolescents. Each year, almost 5,000 teens, ages 15 to 24, kill themselves. The suicide rate for this age group has nearly tripled since 1960.

According to the American Academy of Child and Adolescent Psychiatry, depression and suicidal feelings are treatable emotional conditions. Early recognition and diagnosis along with appropriate treatment are the keys to success.

SUBSTANCE ABUSE

Some teens abuse alcohol and other drugs for a variety of reasons, including curiosity, because it feels good, to manage stress, and to fit in. The research is vague on which teens are likely to experiment but stop before they become addicted and which will develop serious substance abuse issues. The National Institute on Drug Abuse (NIDA) found in 2009, during their annual survey, that overall drug use among teens is declining for most substances. In fact, cigarette use is at its lowest trend ever. However, smokeless tobacco use is on the rise, along with the nonmedical use of prescription drugs.

Teenagers at risk for developing substance abuse issues are those with a family history of substance abuse, those who are depressed, those with low self-esteem, and those who do not feel they fit in.

Teenagers abuse a variety of drugs, both legal and illegal. Legally available drugs include alcohol, prescribed medications, inhalants, and cough, cold, sleep, and diet medications. Illegal drugs commonly abused are marijuana, cocaine, crack, speed, LSD, PCP, opiates, heroin, and Ecstasy.

The reasons that some adolescents develop serious drug problems are many. Among the factors that place adolescents at increased risk are a lack of parental supervision, poor communication between parents and teens, unclear rules for behavior both in and outside the home, and conflict within the family.

NIDA finds that parents and friends can have a positive influence on behavior related to drug and alcohol abuse. In fact, positive family and peer influence can continue as the adolescent or teen grows older. Active parents can not only prevent drug and alcohol abuse with their teen but also can create positive impacts in other areas of their teens' lives. However, the other side of this coin is also true. NIDA finds that negative family and peer relationships can lead to an increase in drug and alcohol use and abuse.

Experts from the National Youth Anti-Drug Media Campaign attempt to educate parents, friends, and teens on how to spot the signs that a teen has a serious problem with drugs. Some items the organization cautions to watch for include: changes in friends; changes in school, such as missing class or failing grades; evidence of drug paraphernalia or drugs; or even borrowing or stealing money or prescription pills. The group mentions, however, that many of these signs and symptoms are also common to being a teen.

Fact Or Fiction?

If I say no to alcohol, I won't fit in.

The Facts: The National Institute on Alcohol Abuse and Alcoholism says that teens often overestimate the numbers of other teens who drink. While resisting the pressure to drink is a real issue for teens, it is easier to refuse than you might think. Experts suggest practicing excuses and how to say "no, thanks." They recommend spending time with friends who do not drink. They also urge teens to stay active and enjoy physical activities, as most drinking occurs when teens are just "hanging out." And finally, they warn against going to parties and other social situations unprepared. A teen has a greater chance of resisting peer pressure and the temptation to drink if he or she has a plan to handle the pressure.

Early recognition and treatment of any of the issues affecting teens and family life are important for both parents and teens. Families should seek help to get the information and resources they need to take appropriate action to restore physical and emotional health.

See also: Arguments and the Family; Communication Styles and Families; Family Boundaries; Family Counseling; Family Rules; Violence and the Family

FURTHER READING

Canfield, Jack, and Kent Healy. *The Success Principles for Teens: How to Get from Where You Are to Where You Want to Be, The Success Principles.* Deerfield Beach, Fla.: HCI, 2008.

Carlson, Dale, and Hannah Carlson. *Addiction: The Brain.* Madison, Conn.: Bick Publishing House, 2010.

■ VIOLENCE AND THE FAMILY

Actions, attitudes, or words that harm or threaten other members of a family. The violence may be directed at a child, partner, parent, spouse, or sibling. It can occur between family members of the same or different generations. Family violence is a widespread problem in the United States, often resulting in emotional and physical harm, and sometimes death.

PHYSICAL AND SEXUAL VIOLENCE

Violence in a family can be physical, sexual, or psychological. It can be directed from an adult to a child, an adult to another adult, or from a sibling to another sibling. **Child abuse** involves physical injury of a child by the adult who is supposed to be the child's caretaker. **Sexual abuse** occurs whenever there is any form of sexual contact between an adult and a child. When violence occurs between adult partners, it is called **intimate partner violence.**

The consequences of abuse are serious and long-lasting. Children who experience violence often suffer life-long psychological consequences, including depression, poor self-esteem, substance abuse, and other mental and emotional problems. During early childhood and adolescence, their development may be slowed or halted. Preschoolers may be anxious, experience nightmares, and display inappropriate sexual behavior. School-age children may be fearful, aggressive, or hyperactive. They may have problems at school, suffer nightmares, experience mental illness, and seem to go backwards in their development in a condition called regressive behavior. Adolescents may become depressed, withdrawn, and suicidal. They may injure themselves, engage in illegal activities, run away from home, and abuse illicit drugs and alcohol.

Fact Or Fiction?

Women don't commit violent acts against their partners.

The Facts: Women are less likely to commit violent acts against their partners than men are, but an increasing number of women are resorting to violence in their disputes with their partners. Still, men and women tend to assault each other in different ways. In the National Violence Against Women Survey, 22.1 percent of women, compared to 7.4 percent of men, said an intimate partner had assaulted them at some point in the relationship.

In 2008, the Centers for Disease Control and Prevention published data collected in 2005 that finds that women experience 2 million injuries from intimate partner violence each year. Almost 25 percent of women in the United States have experienced violence by a current or former spouse or boyfriend at some point in their lives; making it worse, women are much more likely than men to be victimized by a current or former intimate partner. Data regarding spousal abuse indicate that 84 percent of women are victims of spousal abuse, and about three-fourths of the persons who commit family violence are male. During 2007 in the United States, there were 248,300 rapes/sexual assaults reported, which is an increase of more than 500 assaults per day, up from 190,600 in 2005. Rape statistics indicate that women were more likely than men to be victims; the rate for rape/sexual assault for persons age 12 or older in 2007 was 1.8 per 1,000 for females and 0.1 per 1,000 for males. Other data suggest that women are less likely than men to commit severe assaults, such as beating their partner, threatening him with a gun or knife, or using a gun or knife.

Intimate partner violence and child abuse often go hand in hand. Men who are physically violent toward their partners are also likely to be sexually violent and direct that violence toward their children. Adults who experienced or witnessed violence in their families as children are more likely to commit acts of violence toward their partners and children or to become victims of violence.

MEASURING VIOLENCE IN THE FAMILY

In 2007, according to estimates from the National Clearinghouse on Child Abuse and Neglect, an estimated 794,000 children were victims of child abuse and neglect. Of those, more than 59 percent suffered neglect, 10.8 percent were victims of physical abuse, almost 7.6 percent were sexually abused, and seven percent were emotionally maltreated. Many children were victims of more than one type of maltreatment.

About 48 percent of child abuse cases reported in 2007 were male and 52 percent were female. Female children are more likely to be victims of sexual abuse, while males are more likely to be emotionally abused and experience serious physical injuries. More than half of all victims of abuse and neglect are white, 21.7 percent are African American, and 20.8 percent are Latino. Native Americans and Asian Americans account for less than 2.4 percent of reported cases of child maltreatment.

Children who are four years old and younger are the most likely to die as a result of child abuse and neglect. Forty-two percent of children who died as a result of maltreatment in 2007 were younger than a year, while 75.7 percent were under four years of age. Of those, the majority were boys. In 2002, 553 boys and 387 girls died as a result of maltreatment. About 56 percent of fatalities were male children and 44 percent were female. In 2007, 75.7 percent of child fatality victims were younger than four years. Overall, it is estimated that 1,760 children died as the result of neglect or abuse in 2007.

TEENS SPEAK

About a Year Ago, My Father Broke My Arm

I had returned home after seeing a movie with my friends. He had been sitting at home, drinking, while I was at the movie. The minute I opened the door, he started yelling at me about how inconsiderate I was to stay out that late and how much concern I had caused my mother. I ignored him—after all, I had told my mother where I was going and she had said it was okay.

He yelled louder, and I kept ignoring him. I was smearing peanut butter on a piece of bread when I heard him come up behind me. He shoved me into the kitchen counter, so hard that it knocked my breath away. I heard the bones in my forearm snap when I hit the counter.

I knew better. I had learned a long time ago that it is best to disappear when he is on one of his drinking sprees. Anybody who is in the way—my mother, the dog, the cat, or me—is a potential target. Once he even got so angry that he smashed the fish bowl. We had all learned to disappear.

My mother took me to the emergency room. When the nurse asked what happened, I told her that I fell. I couldn't tell her that my father had slammed me into the counter. My mother didn't say anything to the nurse in the emergency room either. I knew why: She had been there before herself, with a broken nose, cracked ribs, and more that she had never told me about.

The next day at school I told my friends I had fallen off my bike. But my math teacher, Mrs. Harding, asked me to stay after school so she could have a word with me. She asked me how I had hurt my arm. When I started to tell the "falling down" story she asked, "How did you get that bruise on your cheek? It sure looks to me like someone hit you. Would you like to talk about it?" That's when I started crying.

I didn't know where to go for help. I talked with Mrs. Harding for a long time that night. She asked me about my family, my dad, and how he treated me. She was the first person who ever used the word *abuse* to me. I had never thought of myself as being abused before. Dad's angry drunken sprees had always been a part of life.

When I got home that night, Dad was furious because I was late and he was waiting for dinner. He slapped me across the face. I could hear Mom crying in the back room. That's when I knew I had to get out of there. I called the number of the domestic violence shelter that Mrs. Harding had given me.

I stayed at the shelter for a week. I moved in with my best friend Bess and her family after that. I started working after school at a fast-food restaurant down the street, and my mother sends me money when she can. In her last letter she said she was saving up so she could get away. I worry about my mom—but I know that she needs to make her own decision to leave. I hope she will. It was the hardest, but best, decision I ever made.

Many experts believe child fatalities due to abuse and neglect are greater than statistics suggest. Because states define key words such as *child homicide, abuse,* and *neglect* differently, the number and types of child fatalities linked to maltreatment vary. In addition, child abuse and neglect may be involved in some deaths that are attributed to accidents, sudden infant death syndrome (SIDS), or other causes.

A study published in *Pediatrics* in 2002, "Under-ascertainment of Child Maltreatment Fatalities by Death Certificates," confirms that these estimates are low. A team of researchers led by Tessa Crume of the Colorado Department of Public Health and Environment compared data on child maltreatment fatalities with information on the death certificates of children who died in Colorado between January 1990 and January 1998. Crume and her colleagues estimate that more than half of children's deaths resulting from abuse or neglect were not recorded.

Almost 56.5 percent of those who maltreat the children they are supposed to be caring for are women, and in 45 percent of cases, the mother acts alone. About 34.5 percent of women and 30 percent of men who maltreat children are younger than 30. In 2007, parents were responsible for 66 percent of neglect, 9.7 percent physical abuse, and 2.4 percent sexual abuse.

Q & A

Question: My father sexually abused me, then told me that he would hurt my mom if I told anyone. What do I do?

Answer: It's common for abusers to try to manipulate their victims into keeping quiet, either by convincing them that the abuse is their own fault or threatening to hurt them or someone they love if they tell. But keeping the abuse a secret doesn't protect anyone. It only allows the abuse to continue. Talk to someone you can trust: a friend's parent, teacher, counselor, doctor, or other adult.

Violence toward children is often linked to violence toward adult intimate partners. According to the Centers for Disease Control and Prevention (CDC), each year a current or former partner or date physically or sexually assaults an estimated 1.5 million women and 835,000 men in the United States. The costs of health care for these incidents is more than $5.8 billion a year. Nearly $4.1 billion is spent on medical and mental health-care services. Although both women and men can be victims of intimate partner violence, estimates from the National Violence Against Women Survey show that one out of four women in the United States has reported a physical assault or rape by an intimate partner, in comparison with one out of 14 men. Women are also more likely than men to be murdered by an intimate partner, with women ages 20 to 29 being at the greatest risk. Ethnicity and race also make a difference. About one out of every three African-American women and one out of every four white women experience intimate partner violence.

Researchers believe that maltreatment of children—including child abuse, sexual abuse, and neglect—and intimate partner violence is far more prevalent than these statistics show. Violence in families often goes unreported, partly because of shame or confusion surrounding such events. Even when incidents are reported, data collection methods may be flawed.

Violence in a family can be physical, sexual, and psychological. Intimate partner violence and child abuse often go hand in hand. Children who are exposed to family violence may experience depression, poor self-esteem, substance abuse, and other mental and emotional problems. When they become adults, they are more likely to commit acts of violence toward their partners and children or to become victims of violence.

While violence does not occur in every family, it is widespread: There are 776,758 children who are victims of maltreatment every year and an estimated 25 percent of women and 8 percent of men are physically or sexually assaulted by a current or former partner or date. Research suggests that both child maltreatment and intimate partner violence are underreported.

See also: Arguments and the Family; Death in the Family; Families, Divided; Teens in Trouble

FURTHER READING

Giardino, Angelo P., and Eileen R. Giardino. *Intimate Partner Violence.* Saint Louis, Mo.: G. W. Medical Publishing, 2009.

Stafford, Ann. *Children Experiencing Domestic Abuse.* Protecting Children and Young People. Edinburgh, Scotland: Dunedin Academic Press, 2010.

HOTLINES AND HELP SITES

Centers for Medicare & Medicaid Services (CMS)
URL: http://www.cms.hhs.gov
Phone: 800-633-4227
Affiliation: The Centers for Medicaid & Medicare Services (CMS) is a federal agency within the U.S. Department of Health and Human Services.
Programs: The CMS administers the Medicare program and works in partnership with states to administer Medicaid, the Children's Health Insurance Program (CHIP), and Health Insurance Portability and Accountability Act (HIPAA) standards. Through Medicare, Medicaid, and CHIP, about one in four Americans receive health care coverage. Nearly 16 million people are covered by Medicare, about 39 million are eligible for Medicaid, and CHIP helps states expand health coverage to as many as 7 million uninsured children.

Children of Lesbians and Gays Everywhere (COLAGE)
URL: http://www.colage.org
Phone: 415-861-5437
Mission: Children of Lesbians and Gays Everywhere (COLAGE) engages, connects, and empowers people to make the world a better place for children of lesbian, gay, bisexual, and transgender parents and families. COLAGE is the only national and international organization in the world specifically supporting young people with gay, lesbian, bisexual, and transgender parents.

Families and Work Institute

URL: http://www.familiesandwork.org

Phone: 212-465-2044

Mission: Families and Work Institute is a nonprofit center for research that provides data to inform decision making on the changing workforce, changing family, and changing community.

Programs: The institute offers some of the most comprehensive research on the U.S. workforce.

Family Caregiver Alliance (FCA)

URL: http://www.caregiver.org

Phone: 415-434-3388

Mission: Founded in 1977, Family Caregiver Alliance (FCA) was the first community-based nonprofit organization in the country to address the needs of families and friends providing long-term care at home.

Programs: FCA now offers programs at national, state, and local levels to support and sustain caregivers. It provides information, education, services, research, and advocacy to support and sustain the important work of families nationwide caring for loved ones with chronic, disabling health conditions.

The Future of Children

URL: http://www.futureofchildren.org

Phone: 609-258-5894

Affiliation: The Future of Children is a publication of the Woodrow Wilson School of Public and International Affairs at Princeton University and the Brookings Institution.

Mission: The Future of Children seeks to promote effective policies and programs for children by providing policy makers, service providers, and the media with timely, objective information based on the best available research.

National Campaign to Prevent Teen Pregnancy

URL: http://www.teenpregnancy.org

Phone: 202-478-8500

Affiliation: The National Campaign to Prevent Teen Pregnancy, founded in February 1996, is a nonprofit, nonpartisan initiative supported almost entirely by private donations.

Mission: The mission of the National Campaign to Prevent Teen Pregnancy is to improve the well-being of children, youths, and families by reducing teen pregnancy. The campaign's goal is to reduce the teen pregnancy rate by one-third between 1996 and 2005.

National Domestic Violence Hotline

URL: http://www.ndvh.org

Phone: 800-799-7233 or 800-787-3224 (TTY)

Programs. The National Domestic Violence Hotline provides victims of domestic violence with a toll-free hotline 24 hours a day, 365 days a year. With a database of more than 4,000 shelters and service providers across the United States, Puerto Rico, Alaska, Hawaii, and the U.S. Virgin Islands, the hotline provides callers with information that they might otherwise have found difficult or impossible to obtain. Bilingual staff and a language line are available for every non-English-speaking caller. Deaf abused women can also find help at the hotline by calling the TTY line.

National Institute on Media and the Family (NIMF)

URL: http://www.mediafamily.org

Phone: 888-672-KIDS (5437)

Mission: The National Institute on Media and the Family (NIMF) maximizes the benefits and minimizes the harm of media on children and families through research, education, and advocacy. Founded by psychologist David Walsh, Ph.D., in 1996, the Institute is a nonprofit, national resource center for research, information, and education about the impact of the media on children and families. The vision of the NIMF is to build healthy families and communities through the wise use of media.

National Network for Child Care (NNCC)

URL: http://www.nncc.org

Affiliation: National Network for Child Care (NNCC) is supported by the Cooperative State Research, Education and Extension Service, U.S. Department of Agriculture, and CYFERNet—the Cooperative Extension System's Children, Youth, and Family Network.

Mission: The NNCC's goal is to share knowledge about children and child care from the vast resources of the land grant universities with parents, professionals, practitioners, and the general public.

Programs: The NNCC unites the expertise of many of the nation's leading universities through the outreach system of cooperative extension. The NNCC Web site offers more than 1,000 publications and resources related to child care, an e-mail listserv, and support and assistance from experts in child care and child development. A newsletter is published four times a year.

Office of Family Assistance (OFA)

URL: http://www.acf.hhs.gov/programs/ofa/dts

Affiliation: The Office of Family Assistance (OFA) is located in the U.S. Department of Health and Human Services, Administration for Children and Families.

Programs: The OFA oversees the Temporary Assistance for Needy Families (TANF) program that was created by the Welfare Reform Law of 1996. TANF became effective July 1, 1997, and replaced what was then commonly known as welfare: Aid to Families with Dependent Children (AFDC) and the Job Opportunities and Basic Skills Training (JOBS) programs. TANF provides assistance and work opportunities to needy families by granting states the federal funds and wide flexibility to develop and implement their own welfare programs.

Office of Foster Care and Adoption (OFCA)

URL: http://www.umassmed.edu/adoption/index/aspx

Phone: 508-856-5397

Affiliation: The Office of Foster Care and Adoption is part of the University of Massachusetts Worcester Campus Center for Adoption Research.

Mission: The mission of the OFCA is to help state agencies and health care organizations optimize the effects of health care initiatives that are intended to provide resources to the underserved.

Programs: The OFCA uses the knowledge and resources of the University of Massachusetts Medical School to develop counseling and service models to advance well-being in the community. Services are provided for public adoption and foster care, medical and behavioral issues, and finding permanent homes for children in foster care.

Office of Foster Care & Adoptive Education & Policy

URL: http://www.centerforadoptionresearch.org

Mission: The Center for Adoption Research is dedicated to developing practical responses to the real world challenges presented by adoption and foster care.

Programs: The center was established in 1996 to study issues related to foster care and adoption. It provides independent research, analysis, and evaluation of adoption and foster care policy and practice. The center is developing professional training programs and resources in disciplines, including medicine, education, social work, policy, and law.

Option Line
URL: http://pregnancycenters.org
Phone: 800-395-HELP (4357)

Programs: Option Line consultants refer each caller to a pregnancy resource center in her area for answers to questions about abortion, pregnancy tests, STDs, adoption, parenting, medical referrals, housing, and many other issues. The toll-free number is available 24 hours a day, seven days a week. Callers from across the country can reach a trained, caring person and then be connected to a pregnancy resource center near them for one-on-one help.

Parents, Families, and Friends of Lesbians and Gays (PFLAG)
URL: http://www.pflag.org
Phone: 202-467-8180

Affiliation: Parents, Families, and Friends of Lesbians and Gays (PFLAG) is a national nonprofit organization with more than 250,000 members and supporters and over 500 affiliates in the United States. This vast grassroots network is cultivated, resourced, and serviced by the PFLAG national office, located in Washington, D.C., the national board of directors, and 14 regional directors.

Mission: To promote the health and well-being of gay, lesbian, bisexual, and transgender persons, their families, and their friends through: support, to cope with an adverse society; education, to enlighten an ill-informed public; and advocacy, to end discrimination and to secure equal civil rights.

Programs: PFLAG provides opportunity for dialogue about sexual orientation and gender identity and acts to create a society that is healthy and respectful of human diversity.

Parents Without Partners

URL: http://www.parentswithoutpartners.org

Phone: 800-637-7974

Mission: Parents Without Partners provides single parents and their children with an opportunity for enhancing personal growth, self-confidence, and sensitivity toward others by offering an environment for support, friendship, and the exchange of parenting techniques.

TeenGrowth.com

URL: http://www.teengrowth.com

Programs: TeenGrowth focuses exclusively on the educational health issues of adolescents. The site provides a secure environment where teens can ask questions and find reliable and useful information about subjects such as emotions, peer pressure, drugs, alcohol, puberty, sex, fitness, and stress. The Medical Advisory Board, comprising well-known and respected physicians in the pediatric community, oversees all content on the site, thereby guaranteeing its medical accuracy.

U.S. Department of Housing and Urban Development (HUD)

URL: http://www.hud.gov

Phone: 202-708-1112; 202-708-1455

Affiliation: HUD is a federal agency.

Mission: HUD's mission is to increase homeownership, support community development, and increase access to affordable housing free from discrimination. To fulfill this mission, HUD will embrace high standards of ethics, management and accountability and forge new partnerships—particularly with faith-based and community organizations—that leverage resources and improve HUD's ability to be effective on the community level.

GLOSSARY

abandonment   the refusal of a parent to physically, emotionally, or financially support his or her child

Activities of Daily Living (ADL)   the scale used to measure a person's ability to perform physical tasks

adolescence   the stage of growth and development between childhood and adulthood entailing major physical, cognitive, emotional, and social changes

adoptive parents   adults who assume parental rights and responsibilities for a child not related by birth

alimony   payment to or from a former spouse as part of a separation or divorce agreement

Alzheimer's disease   a progressive, degenerative brain disorder

artificial insemination   a process by which pregnancy is achieved without sexual intercourse

assets   the monetary resources of an individual, family, or business

bereavement   sadness about the loss of a loved one

bias   prejudice

birth families   biological parents and siblings

bisexual   being sexually attracted to both men and women

celibate   abstaining from sexual intercourse

child abuse   physical or emotional injury of a child

child support   money paid by a parent to help support children not living with him or her

cohabitation   the practice of living together without marriage

common-pot method and the two-pot method   common economic patterns used by blended families to benefit and raise the children according to their needs

community property states   states in which all property obtained during the marriage—other than a gift or inheritance—belongs equally to both spouses

companionate family   a family which is seen as the primary source of emotional satisfaction and personal happiness

compromise   a mutually acceptable solution that is not exactly what either party to a dispute wanted but is fair and can meet each person's minimum needs

custody   legal responsibility for the care and protection of a child

debt   an amount owed to another

depression   overwhelming feeling of sadness and grief

domestic partners   a stable, intimate relationship between two people who are financially interdependent

dual earner   a family in which both spouses are part of the labor force

dysfunctions   abnormal or unhealthy behaviors or interactions

economic parity   earning the same pay for performing the same work

effective preferences   the actions people take when they focus on broad concerns, such as the long-term consequences of their actions and the implications for others

egalitarian   characterized by an arrangement of equality in a marriage

ejaculation   the expulsion of seminal fluid from the penis at the climax of sexual excitement; the fluid contains spermatozoa, which can fertilize an ovum for reproduction

emancipate   to legally release a child from the control of a parent or guardian

erections   occurrences during male sexual arousal, which involve blood flowing into the penis, making it firm

estrangement   alienation of family members from each other due to unresolved conflict

ethnicity   the cultural heritage of a particular group

exit   an actively destructive response in a family in which the offended person leaves, threatens to end the relationship, or engages in abusive acts such as yelling or hitting

fertile   the ability to produce healthy eggs and sperm for reproduction

fertility rate   the average number of children a woman has in her lifetime

fetus   the unborn baby from the eighth week after fertilization to birth

foster parents   persons licensed to care for a child by the government or a social service agency

gene biological unit that directs production of a particular protein and determines the presence or absence of a particular trait

genetic passed down from ancestor to ancestor, and referring to characteristics of an individual based on inherited qualities, such as eye and hair color

given preferences the actions people take when they focus on short-term, self-centered, immediate reactions to an event

guardianship a legal proceeding by which a court appoints an individual to assume the care of a person who is unable to care for himself or herself

heterosexual being attracted to people of the opposite sex

homosexual being attracted to people of the same sex

hormone a chemical substance that some cells in the body release to help other cells work; for example, insulin is a hormone that helps the body use glucose as energy

immune response the reaction of a person's body to an irritant

income tax a tax on earnings payable to city, state, and/or federal governments

integrative agreements creative ways worked out to resolve problems and restore peace

intercountry adoptions international adoptions

interracial marriage a marriage in which the husband and wife are of different races

intimate partner violence violence between adult partners in a relationship

joint custody custody arrangements in which parents share physical and legal custody

legal custody custody arrangements that determine who will make decisions about how a child is raised

logrolling making concessions on one issue if the other person will make concessions on another, while still maintaining commitment to one's central goals

long-term care health services provided to people with chronic conditions, physical disabilities, and/or cognitive impairment

mediator a person who usually has a background in law or the behavioral sciences and specializes in helping couples resolve the issues that arise in a divorce

Medicaid a federal-state program that provides health-care assistance to low-income people

Medicare a federal health insurance program for people 65 and over and certain disabled people under 65

menstruation the loss of blood and tissue lining the uterus each month a woman does not become pregnant

monogamous description of couples who engage in sex only with each other

mons veneris the fatty tissue covering the female pubic bone

next-of-kin a person's closest living relative either by blood or by marriage

obstetrician a physician who specializes in delivering babies

parenting coalition an arrangement in which the divorced and remarried biological parents and the stepparents cooperate in rearing their biological children and stepchildren

parenting coordinator a person who works within the structure of a couple's divorce decree to help parents settle disagreement about children

paternity   identification of the father of a child

penis   the male organ, made up of nerves, blood vessels, and spongy and fibrous tissue

pension payments   income received upon retirement

perpetrator   a person who commits an offensive action

physical custody   custody arrangements that define where the child will live

physical dependence   the physical craving for and the compulsive use of a substance despite harmful psychological, physical, or social consequences

postpartum depression   women's experiences of depression shortly after giving birth

power of attorney   a legal document that authorizes another person to act on one's behalf

premenstrual syndrome (PMS)   a group of symptoms some women experience just prior to menstruation; the symptoms may include irritability, insomnia, fatigue, anxiety, depression, headache, water retention, and/or abdominal pain or cramps

prenatal care   medical care during pregnancy

prenuptial agreement   a legal agreement arranged prior to marriage stating who owns property acquired before marriage and, during the marriage, and how property will be divided in the event of divorce

profit sharing   a plan in which employers share their profits with employees at the employer's discretion

reconstituted families   another term for blended families

ripple effect   the way some actions can have a spreading, and usually unintentional, influence, in the same way that ripples expand outward on water when a pebble is dropped into a pond

role models   people who are considered worthy of imitation

scrotum   the pouch of skin that holds the testes

separation   a couple's decision to live apart by mutual agreement or under a court order

sexual abuse   any form of sexual contact between an adult and a child

sexually transmitted disease (STD)   communicable disease transmitted by sexual intercourse or genital contact

sexual orientation   a person's romantic, emotional, or sexual attraction to a person of the opposite sex and/or one's own sex

sexual phenomena   developments in males and females, both physical and emotional, that are the result of the ability to reproduce during adolescence

sibling   a brother or sister

sibling rivalry   competition between brothers and sisters for their parents' attention, approval, and affection

social isolation   loneliness due to a lack of a social network of friends and acquaintances

sole custody   custody arrangements that legally establish care by one parent

staff ratio   the number of children in a day care situation related to the number of staff to care for them

stepfamilies   families formed by parents' subsequent marriages

stereotype   an oversimplified generalization about a group of people

testes   the paired male organs that produce sperm and male hormones

transracial adoption   the adoption of a child of one race by parents of another

transsexual   showing a strong desire to live one's life as a member of the opposite sex

uterus   a hollow female organ where the fetus develops

visitation rights   the legal right to spend time with one's child

wills   legal documents expressing a person's wishes regarding the disposal of his or her property after death

INDEX

Boldface page numbers indicate extensive treatment of a topic.